UNIVERSITY OF BIRMINGHAM
BARNES MEDICAL LIBRARY

D1336920

COLOR ATLAS OF

FOOT & ANKLE ANATOMY

Second Edition

Robert M H McMinn MD, PhD, FRCS (Eng.)
Emeritus Professor of Anatomy
Royal College of Surgeons of England
and University of London
London, UK

Ralph T Hutchings
Freelance Photographer
Formerly Chief Medical Laboratory Scientific Officer
Royal College of Surgeons of England
London, UK

Bari M Logan MA, FMA, Hon. MBIE
University Prosector
Department of Anatomy
University of Cambridge
Cambridge, UK

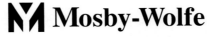

London Baltimore Barcelona Bogotá Boston Buenos Aires Caracas Carlsbad, CA Chicago Madrid Mexico City Milan Naples, FL New York
Philadelphia St. Louis Seoul Singapore Sydney Taipei Tokyo Toronto Wiesbaden

Project Managers:	Jane Hurd-Cosgrave
	Dave Burin
Developmental Editor:	Lucy Hamilton
Designer:	Ian Spick
Layout Artist:	Jonathan Brenchley
Cover Design:	Kevin Palmer
	Rob Curran
Illustration:	Marion Tasker
Publisher:	Geoff Greenwood

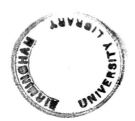

Copyright © 1996 Times Mirror International Publishers Limited

Published by Mosby-Wolfe, an imprint of Times Mirror International Publishers Limited

Printed in Spain by Grafos S.A. Arte sobre papel, Barcelona, Spain

ISBN 0 7234 1995 7

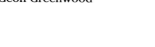

All rights reserved. No part of this publication may be reproduced, stored in a retrieval system, copied or transmitted, in any form or by any means, electronic, mechanical, photocopying, recording or otherwise without written permission from the Publisher or in accordance with the provisions of the Copyright Act 1988, or under the terms of any licence permitting limited copying issued by the Copyright Licensing Agency, 33–34 Alfred Place, London, WC1E 7DP.

Any person who does any unauthorised act in relation to this publication may be liable to criminal prosecution and civil claims for damages.

Permission to photocopy or reproduce solely for internal or personal use is permitted for libraries or other users registered with the Copyright Clearance Center, provided that the base fee of $4.00 per chapter plus $.10 per page is paid directly to the Copyright Clearance Center, 21 Congress Street, Salem, MA 01970. This consent does not extend to other kinds of copying, such as copying for general distribution, for advertising or promotional purposes, for creating new collected works, or for resale.

For full details of all Times Mirror International Publishers Limited titles, please write to Times Mirror International Publishers Limited, Lynton House, 7–12 Tavistock Square, London WC1H 9LB, England.

A CIP catalogue record for this book is available from the British Library.

Library of Congress Cataloging-in-Publication Data has been applied for.

Preface

The scope of this new edition has been extended to include other features of the lower limb, with emphasis on the major joints - the hip and the knee - in view of their close association with the function of the foot. In addition to new notes, every dissection has a commentary, explaining what has been displayed and drawing attention to the most important features. There are new radiographs and images, as well as an enlarged Appendix, with some details of local anaesthesia of the foot and new diagrams of muscles, nerves and vessels.

We hope that the atlas will continue to find particular favour with podiatrists and chiropodists, and all who have an interest in the form and function of the lower limb.

Acknowledgements

For the provision of radiographs and images we are grateful to Dr Peter Abrahams, Dr Oscar Craig, Dr Kate Stevens and Mr W Stripp; they are acknowledged on the appropriate pages.

We would also like to thank Dave Burin of Times Mirror International Publishers for sorting out many editorial details, and Dr David Johnson for proof-reading.

Contents

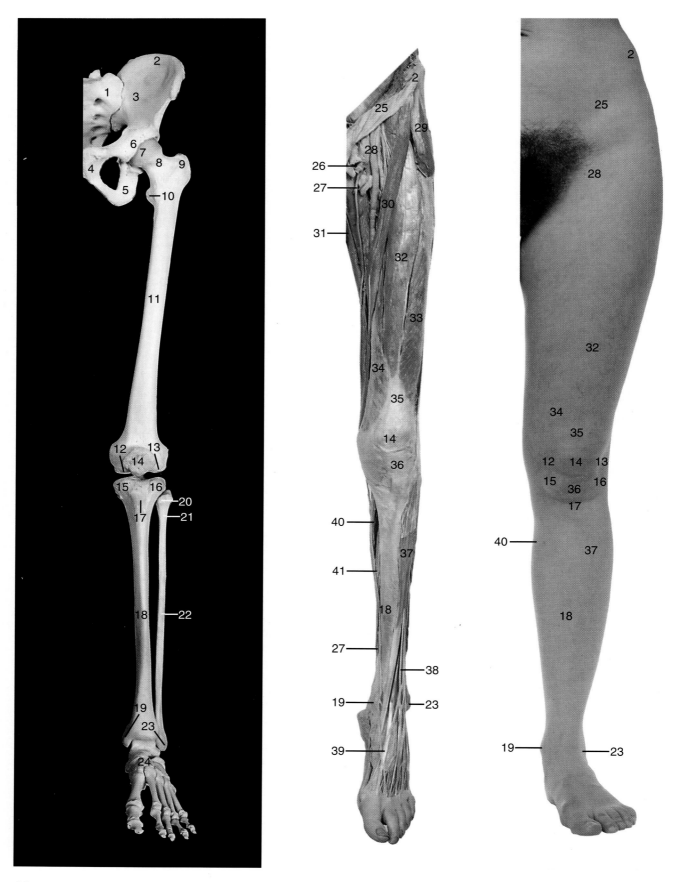

LOWER LIMB SURVEY
Bones, muscles and surface landmarks of the left lower limb, from the front

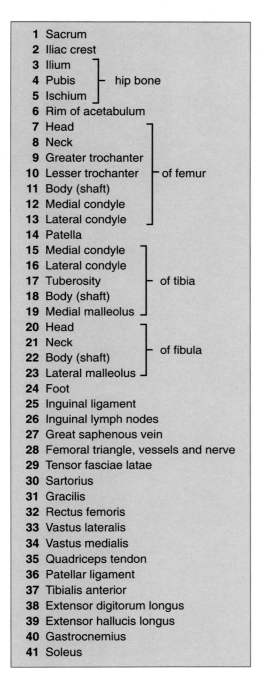

 1 Sacrum
 2 Iliac crest
 3 Ilium ⎤
 4 Pubis ⎬ hip bone
 5 Ischium ⎦
 6 Rim of acetabulum
 7 Head ⎤
 8 Neck │
 9 Greater trochanter │
10 Lesser trochanter ⎬ of femur
11 Body (shaft) │
12 Medial condyle │
13 Lateral condyle ⎦
14 Patella
15 Medial condyle ⎤
16 Lateral condyle │
17 Tuberosity ⎬ of tibia
18 Body (shaft) │
19 Medial malleolus ⎦
20 Head ⎤
21 Neck │
22 Body (shaft) ⎬ of fibula
23 Lateral malleolus ⎦
24 Foot
25 Inguinal ligament
26 Inguinal lymph nodes
27 Great saphenous vein
28 Femoral triangle, vessels and nerve
29 Tensor fasciae latae
30 Sartorius
31 Gracilis
32 Rectus femoris
33 Vastus lateralis
34 Vastus medialis
35 Quadriceps tendon
36 Patellar ligament
37 Tibialis anterior
38 Extensor digitorum longus
39 Extensor hallucis longus
40 Gastrocnemius
41 Soleus

- The main parts or regions of the lower limb are the gluteal region (consisting of the hip at the side and the buttock at the back), the thigh, the knee, the leg, the ankle and the foot. The term *leg* properly refers to the part between the knee and the foot, although it is commonly used for the whole lower limb.

- The hip bone consists of three bones fused together – the ilium, ischium and pubis – and forms a pelvic girdle. The two hip bones or girdles unite with each other in front at the pubic symphysis, and at the back they join the sacrum at the sacro-iliac joints, so forming the bony pelvis.

- The femur is the bone of the thigh; the tibia and fibula are the bones of the leg.

- The acetabulum of the hip bone and the head of the femur form the hip joint.

- The condyles of the femur and tibia together with the patella form the knee joint.

- The head of the fibula forms a small joint with the tibia, the superior tibiofibular joint. The inferior tibiofibular joint, properly called the tibiofibular syndesmosis (a type of fibrous joint) is a fibrous union between the tibia and fibula just above the ankle joint.

- The ankle is the lower part of the leg in the region of the ankle joint.

- The lower ends of the tibia and fibula articulate with the talus of the foot to form the ankle joint.

- The body of a long bone is commonly called the shaft.

- The adjective 'peroneal' (Greek, see page 39) is now being replaced by the Latin 'fibular' for various vessels and nerves, e.g. common fibular nerve instead of common peroneal nerve, but the older and more familiar 'peroneal' is retained throughout this book.

For details of limb muscles, nerves and arteries see the Appendix:
Muscles – pages 103–109, including **Figs 1–6**.
Nerves – pages 110–112, including **Figs 7–10**.
Arteries – pages 113 and 114, including **Figs. 11** and **12**.

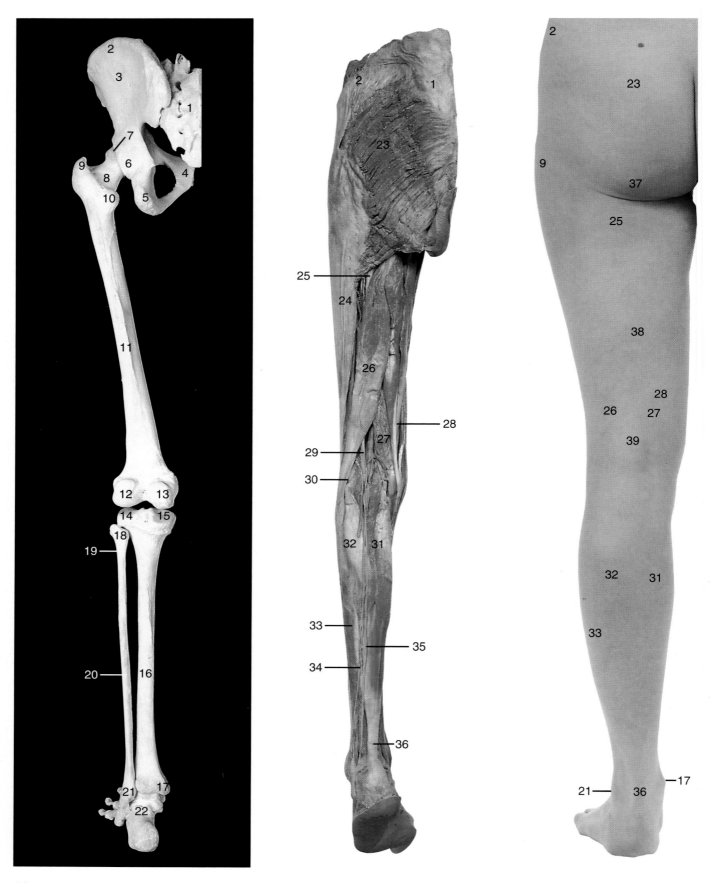

LOWER LIMB SURVEY
Bones, muscles and surface landmarks of the left lower limb, from behind

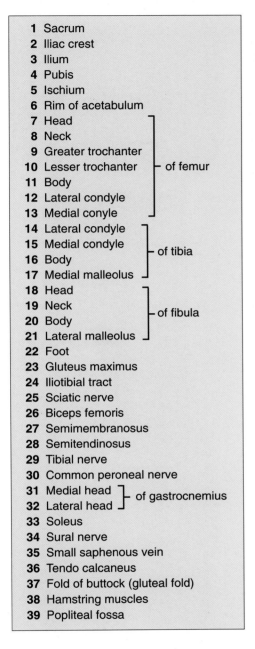

1 Sacrum
2 Iliac crest
3 Ilium
4 Pubis
5 Ischium
6 Rim of acetabulum
7 Head ⎤
8 Neck │
9 Greater trochanter │
10 Lesser trochanter ⎬ of femur
11 Body │
12 Lateral condyle │
13 Medial conyle ⎦
14 Lateral condyle ⎤
15 Medial condyle ⎬ of tibia
16 Body │
17 Medial malleolus ⎦
18 Head ⎤
19 Neck ⎬ of fibula
20 Body │
21 Lateral malleolus ⎦
22 Foot
23 Gluteus maximus
24 Iliotibial tract
25 Sciatic nerve
26 Biceps femoris
27 Semimembranosus
28 Semitendinosus
29 Tibial nerve
30 Common peroneal nerve
31 Medial head ⎤ of gastrocnemius
32 Lateral head ⎦
33 Soleus
34 Sural nerve
35 Small saphenous vein
36 Tendo calcaneus
37 Fold of buttock (gluteal fold)
38 Hamstring muscles
39 Popliteal fossa

- The curved fold of the buttock (**37**) does not correspond to the straight (but oblique) lower border of gluteus maximus (**23**).

- The tendons of gastrocnemius (**31** and **32**) and soleus (**33**) join to form the tendo calcaneus (**36**), known commonly as the Achilles' tendon.

- The muscles on the back of the thigh with prominent tendons – semimembranosus (**27**), semitendinosus (**28**) and biceps femoris (long head, **26**) – are known commonly as the hamstrings (see the note on page 25).

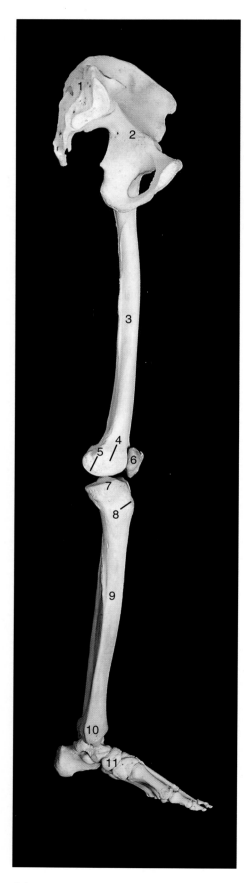

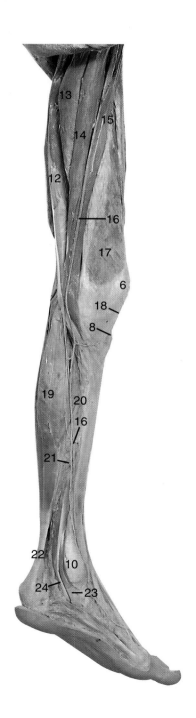

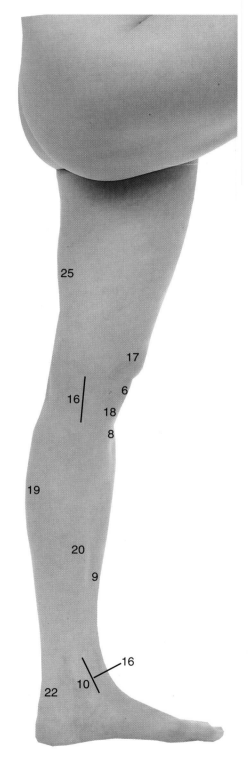

LOWER LIMB SURVEY
Bones, muscles and surface landmarks of the left lower limb, from the medial side

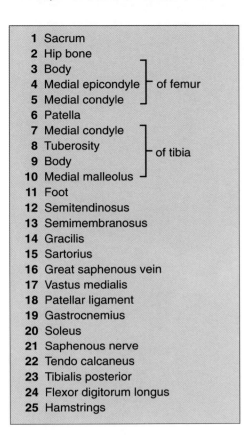

1 Sacrum
2 Hip bone
3 Body ⎤
4 Medial epicondyle ⎬ of femur
5 Medial condyle ⎦
6 Patella
7 Medial condyle ⎤
8 Tuberosity ⎬ of tibia
9 Body ⎥
10 Medial malleolus ⎦
11 Foot
12 Semitendinosus
13 Semimembranosus
14 Gracilis
15 Sartorius
16 Great saphenous vein
17 Vastus medialis
18 Patellar ligament
19 Gastrocnemius
20 Soleus
21 Saphenous nerve
22 Tendo calcaneus
23 Tibialis posterior
24 Flexor digitorum longus
25 Hamstrings

- At the ankle the great saphenous vein (**16**), the longest vein in the body, passes upwards in front of the medial malleolus (**10**). At the knee it lies a hands breadth behind the medial border of the patella (**6**). It ends by draining into the femoral vein (page 22, **12** and **18**).

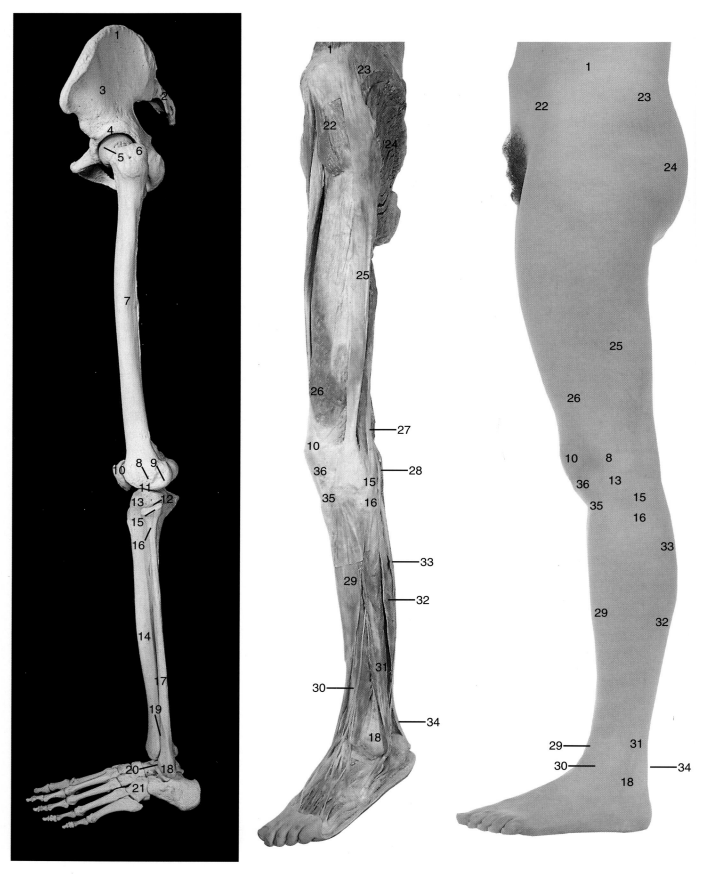

LOWER LIMB SURVEY
Bones, muscles and surface landmarks of the left lower limb, from the lateral side

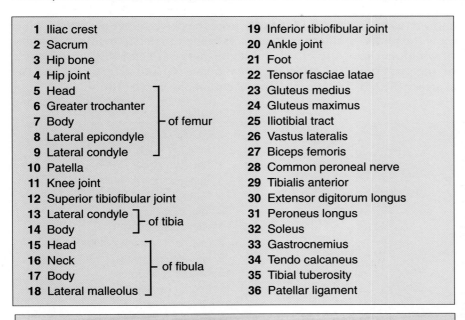

1 Iliac crest	19 Inferior tibiofibular joint
2 Sacrum	20 Ankle joint
3 Hip bone	21 Foot
4 Hip joint	22 Tensor fasciae latae
5 Head ⎤	23 Gluteus medius
6 Greater trochanter ⎥	24 Gluteus maximus
7 Body ⎬ of femur	25 Iliotibial tract
8 Lateral epicondyle ⎥	26 Vastus lateralis
9 Lateral condyle ⎦	27 Biceps femoris
10 Patella	28 Common peroneal nerve
11 Knee joint	29 Tibialis anterior
12 Superior tibiofibular joint	30 Extensor digitorum longus
13 Lateral condyle ⎤ of tibia	31 Peroneus longus
14 Body ⎦	32 Soleus
15 Head ⎤	33 Gastrocnemius
16 Neck ⎥ of fibula	34 Tendo calcaneus
17 Body ⎥	35 Tibial tuberosity
18 Lateral malleolus ⎦	36 Patellar ligament

- The common peroneal nerve (**28**), the only *palpable* major nerve of the lower limb, can be felt as it passes downwards and forwards across the neck of the fibula (**16**).

GLUTEAL REGION
A Sciatic nerve and other gluteal structures of the right side

Most of gluteus maximus (**1**) has been removed (as have the veins that accompany arteries) to show the underlying structures, the most important of which is the sciatic nerve (**14** and **15**). The key to the region is the piriformis muscle (**2**): the superior gluteal artery (**3**) and nerve (**4**) emerge from the pelvis above piriformis, while all other structures leave the pelvis below piriformis. Apart from the sciatic nerve (**14** and **15**), these include the inferior gluteal nerve (**6**) and artery (**22**) and the posterior femoral cutaneous nerve (**16**).

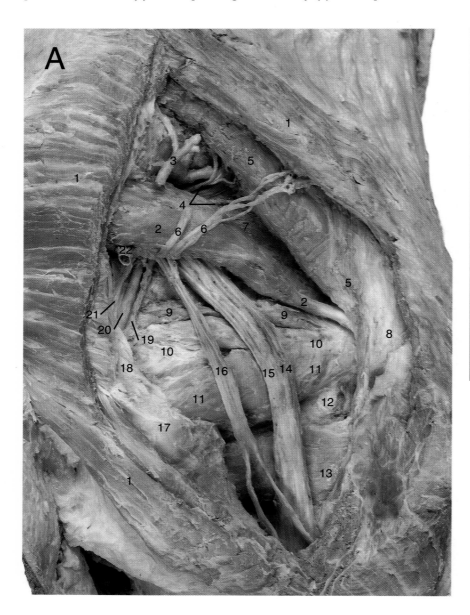

1	Gluteus maximus
2	Piriformis
3	Superior gluteal artery
4	Superior gluteal nerve
5	Gluteus medius
6	Inferior gluteal nerve
7	Gluteus minimus
8	Greater trochanter of femur
9	Superior gemellus
10	Obturator internus
11	Inferior gemellus
12	Obturator externus
13	Quadratus femoris
14	Common peroneal ⎤ part of
15	Tibial ⎦ sciatic nerve
16	Posterior femoral cutaneous nerve
17	Ischial tuberosity
18	Sacrotuberous ligament
19	Nerve to obturator internus
20	Internal pudendal artery
21	Pudendal nerve
22	Inferior gluteal artery

GLUTEAL REGION
B Surface features of the right gluteal region

The interrupted white lines divide the gluteal region into four quadrants. The surface marking of the lower border of piriformis (the dotted white line) is on a line drawn from the midpoint between the posterior superior iliac spine (**9**) and the coccyx (**7**) to the top of the greater trochanter of the femur (**3**). From the midpoint of this line, a curved line (convex laterally) to midway between the ischial tuberosity (**6**) and the greater trochanter (**3**) indicates the course of the upper part of the sciatic nerve, indicated here in yellow.

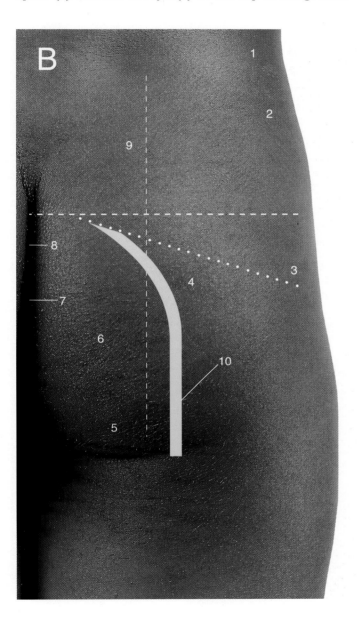

1 Iliac crest
2 Gluteus medius
3 Greater trochanter of femur
4 Gluteus maximus
5 Fold of buttock
6 Ischial tuberosity
7 Tip of coccyx
8 Natal cleft
9 Posterior superior iliac spine
10 Sciatic nerve

- The superior gluteal nerve runs between gluteus medius and minimus and ends in tensor fasciae latae, supplying all three muscles.

- The inferior gluteal nerve passes straight back into gluteus maximus, supplying that muscle only.

- In the gluteal region the sciatic nerve is a flattened band about 1 cm broad. Its two parts (**A14** and **15**) are usually closely bound together in the gluteal region and the back of the thigh (page 25, **B10**). In the popliteal fossa at the back of the knee (page 30, **A**) they separate into the common peroneal nerve, which supplies the front of the leg and dorsum of the foot, and the tibial nerve, which supplies the back of the leg and sole of the foot.

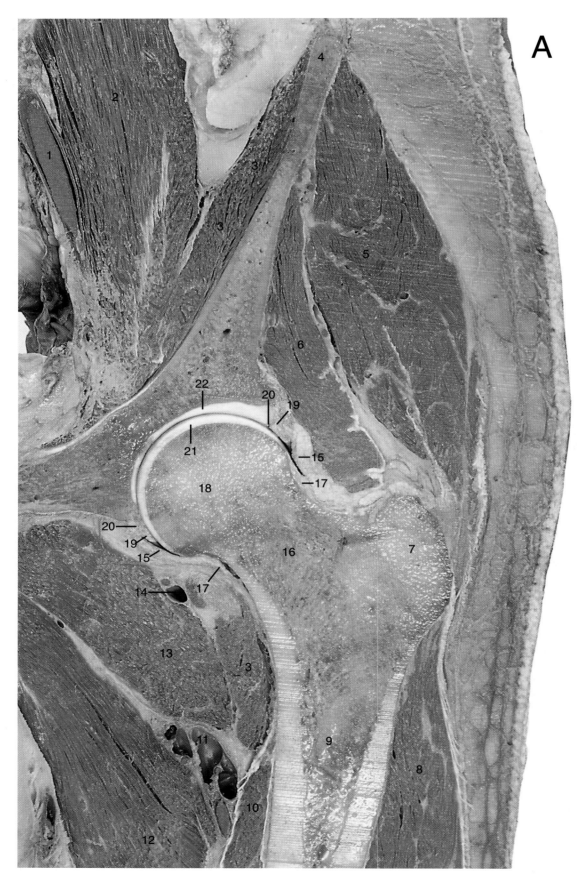

A

HIP JOINT
A Coronal section of the left hip joint, from the front
B Radiograph

The head of the femur (**18**) sits in the hip bone's acetabulum (**20**) which is deepened at the periphery by the fibrous acetabular labrum (**19**). Note the hyaline cartilage on the joint surfaces (**21** and **22**), and the capsule (**15**) whose circular fibres (zona orbicularis, **17**) keep it close to the neck of the femur (**16**). Gluteus medius (**5**) and gluteus minimus (**6**) converge on to the greater trochanter (**7**), and below the head and neck of the femur (**18** and **16**) the tendon of psoas major (**2**) and some muscle fibres of iliacus (**3**) are passing backwards to reach the lesser trochanter on the back of the bone. Compare major features in the section with the radiograph.

1	External iliac artery
2	Psoas major
3	Iliacus
4	Iliac crest
5	Gluteus medius
6	Gluteus minimus
7	Greater trochanter of femur
8	Vastus lateralis
9	Shaft of femur
10	Vastus medialis
11	Profunda femoris vessels
12	Adductor longus
13	Pectineus
14	Medial circumflex femoral vessels
15	Capsule of hip joint
16	Neck of femur
17	Zona orbicularis of capsule
18	Head of femur
19	Acetabular labrum
20	Rim of acetabulum
21	Hyaline cartilage of head
22	Hyaline cartilage of acetabulum
23	Lesser trochanter of femur

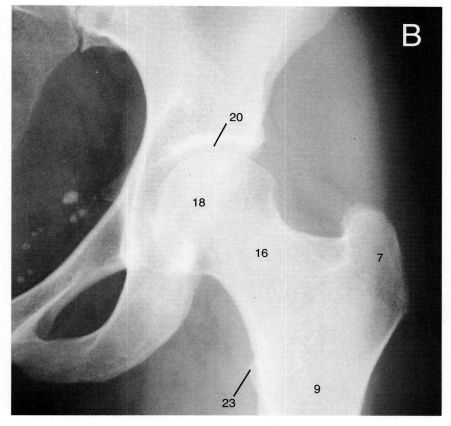

By courtesy of Dr Oscar Craig

- Muscles producing movements at the hip joint:
  Flexion (moving the thigh forwards and upwards towards the abdomen): psoas and iliacus, with rectus femoris, sartorius, tensor fasciae latae, pectineus, adductor longus and adductor brevis.
  Extension (moving the thigh backwards): gluteus maximus, semimembranosus, semitendinosus, long head of biceps and ischial part of adductor magnus.
  Abduction (moving the thigh laterally away from the midline): gluteus medius, gluteus minimus, with tensor fasciae latae and piriformis.
  Adduction (moving the thigh medially towards the midline): adductor longus, adductor brevis, adductor magnus, pectineus, gracilis, quadratus femoris.
  Medial rotation (rotating the thigh inwards in the long axis of the limb): anterior fibres of gluteus medius and gluteus minimus, with tensor fasciae latae. (Electromyography does not support the long-held view that psoas major is a medial rotator.)
  Lateral rotation (rotating the thigh outwards in the long axis of the limb): obturator externus, obturator internus and gemelli, piriformis, quadratus femoris, gluteus maximus and sartorius.

- The coronal section of the joint in **A** demonstrates the thickness of the capsule (**15**) but does not of course show the ligaments that reinforce the outside of the capsule (iliofemoral at the front, and pubofemoral and ischiofemoral below and behind).

THIGH
Front of the right upper thigh
A Inguinal and femoral regions, in the female

Part of the fascia lata (deep fascia of the thigh, **14**) has been removed to display the femoral vessels and nerve and the adjacent muscles. The femoral nerve (**21**), artery (**20**), vein (**18**) and canal (**17**) lie in that order from lateral to medial beneath the inguinal ligament (**19**). The great saphenous vein (**12**) passes through the saphenous opening (**16**) in the fascia lata to enter the femoral vein (**18**); a number of smaller veins enter the great saphenous just before it joins the femoral.

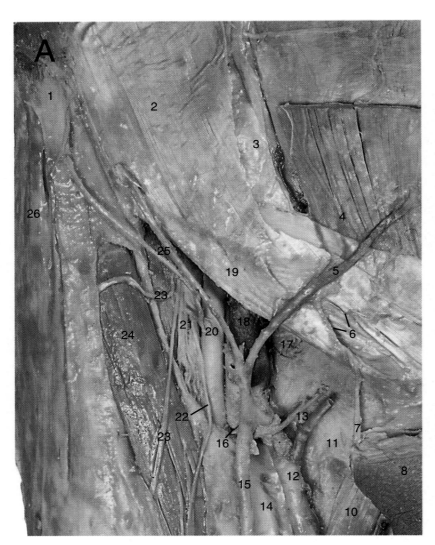

1 Anterior superior iliac spine
2 External oblique aponeurosis
3 Cut edge of rectus sheath
4 Rectus abdominis
5 Superficial epigastric vein
6 Superficial inguinal ring
7 Round ligament of uterus
8 Mons pubis
9 Gracilis
10 Adductor longus
11 Pectineus
12 Great saphenous vein
13 Superficial external pudendal vessels
14 Fascia lata
15 Accessory saphenous vein
16 Lower edge of saphenous opening
17 Position of femoral canal
18 Femoral vein
19 Inguinal ligament
20 Femoral artery
21 Femoral nerve
22 Medial   ⎤ femoral
23 Intermediate ⎦ cutaneous nerve
24 Sartorius
25 Superficial circumflex iliac vessels
26 Fascia lata overlying tensor fasciae
   latae

- The femoral pulse can be felt midway between the anterior superior iliac spine and the midline pubic symphysis (the midinguinal point or femoral point).

- Various superficial veins (**5,13,15,25**) run into the great saphenous vein (**12**); this helps to distinguish the great saphenous from the femoral vein (**18**), which superficially at this level receives only the great saphenous itself. See page 66 for further details of the great saphenous vein.

- Although arising at the *front* of the thigh, the profunda femoris artery is the main supply to muscles on the *back* of the thigh as well as those on the front.

- The adductor canal, which is triangular in cross section, is bounded in front by sartorius, laterally by vastus medialis, and behind by adductor longus (above) and adductor magnus (below). The contents of the adductor canal are the femoral artery and vein, the saphenous nerve and the nerve to vastus medialis.

THIGH
Front of the right upper thigh
B Femoral vessels and nerve, in the male

In this deeper dissection the removal of part of sartorius (**3**) displays the profunda femoris artery (**24**). The femoral artery (**9**) passes in front of adductor longus (**18**); the profunda (**24**) passes behind it. Separation of the adjacent borders of pectineus (**13**) and adductor longus (**18**) allows the anterior division of the obturator nerve (**15**) to be seen in front of adductor brevis (**17**). The medial circumflex femoral artery (**12**) disappears backwards between pectineus (**13**) and the tendon of psoas (hidden behind the uppermost part of the femoral artery (upper **9**). The lateral circumflex femoral artery (**11**, which often arises directly from the femoral artery, as here, and not from the profunda), courses laterally and supplies adjacent muscles. Branches of the femoral nerve (**8**) include the saphenous nerve (**25**) which will run as far as the medial side of the foot.

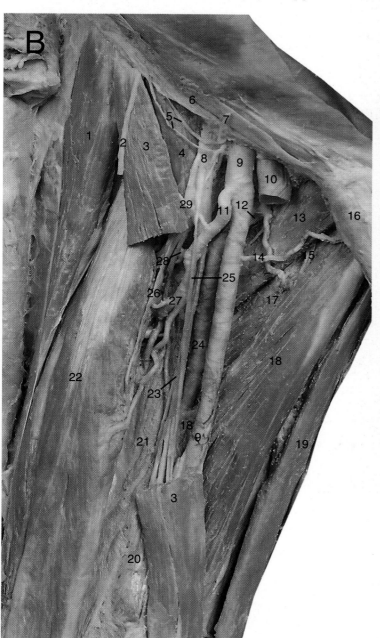

1	Tensor fasciae latae
2	Lateral femoral cutaneous nerve
3	Sartorius
4	Iliacus
5	Superficial circumflex iliac artery (double)
6	Inguinal ligament
7	Superficial epigastric artery
8	Femoral nerve
9	Femoral artery
10	Femoral vein
11	Lateral circumflex femoral artery
12	Medial circumflex femoral artery
13	Pectineus
14	Superficial external pudendal artery
15	Anterior branch of obturator nerve
16	Spermatic cord
17	Adductor brevis
18	Adductor longus
19	Gracilis
20	Vastus medialis
21	Vastus intermedius
22	Rectus femoris
23	Nerve to vastus medialis
24	Profunda femoris artery
25	Saphenous nerve
26	Nerve to rectus femoris
27	Descending ⎤ branch of
28	Transverse ⊢ lateral circumflex
29	Ascending ⎦ femoral artery

THIGH
Lower right thigh
A From the front and medial side

The lower part of sartorius (3) has been displaced medially to open up the lower part of the adductor canal and expose the femoral artery (4) passing through the opening in adductor magnus (6) to enter the popliteal fossa behind the knee and become the popliteal artery.

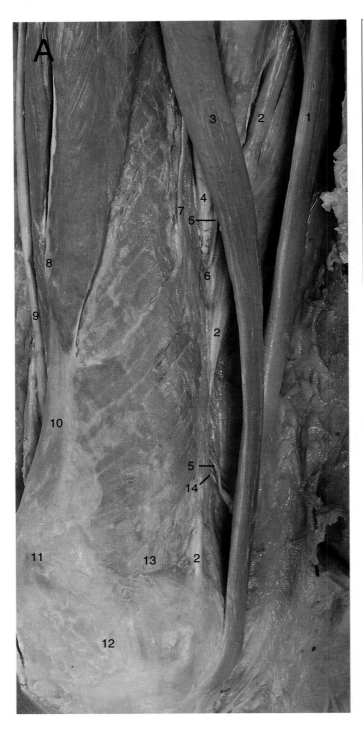

1	Gracilis
2	Adductor magnus
3	Sartorius
4	Femoral artery
5	Saphenous nerve
6	Opening in adductor magnus
7	Vastus medialis and nerve
8	Rectus femoris
9	Iliotibial tract
10	Quadriceps tendon
11	Patella
12	Medial patellar retinaculum
13	Lowest (horizontal) fibres of vastus medialis
14	Saphenous branch of descending genicular artery

THIGH
Lower right thigh
B Cross section at the level of the opening in adductor magnus

The section is viewed as when looking upwards from knee to hip. The three vastus muscles (**1**, **3** and **5**) envelop the femur (**2**) at the front and sides, and rectus femoris (**4**) at this level is narrow and is becoming tendinous. The femoral vessels (**20**) are between vastus medialis (**1**) and adductor magnus (**12**), approaching the adductor magnus opening (**13**), and the profunda femoris vessels (**11**) lie close to the back of the femur (**2**). The sciatic nerve (**10**) is deeply placed between biceps (**8** and **9**) laterally and semimembranosus (**14**) and semitendinosus (**15**) medially.

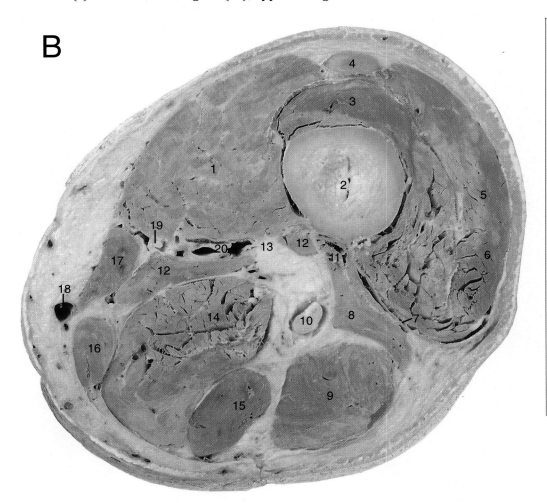

B

1	Vastus medialis
2	Femur
3	Vastus intermedius
4	Rectus femoris
5	Vastus lateralis
6	Iliotibial tract
7	Lateral intermuscular septum
8	Short head of biceps
9	Long head of biceps
10	Sciatic nerve
11	Profunda femoris vessels
12	Adductor magnus
13	Opening in adductor magnus
14	Semimembranosus
15	Semitendinosus
16	Gracilis
17	Sartorius
18	Great saphenous vein
19	Saphenous nerve
20	Femoral vessels

- The muscles commonly called the hamstrings span both the hip and knee joints: they arise from the ischial tuberosity and run to the upper end of the tibia and fibula, and consist of semitendinosus, semimembranosus, and the long head of biceps. The short head of biceps is not a hamstring, since although it joins the long head it arises from the back of the femur and hence does not span the hip joint. Semitendinosus is named from the long tendon at its lower end. Semimembranosus is named from the broad tendinous origin at its upper end.

KNEE JOINT

Left knee joint
A Bones, with the knee joint in extension, from the front
B Bones and ligaments, with the knee joint in flexion and the patella removed, from the front
C Coronal magnetic resonance (MR) image
D Opened up from the front, with the knee joint in extension and the patella turned laterally

Flexion of the knee, as in **B**, exposes a much larger area of the femoral condyles (**4** and **7**) than is seen in extension (as in **A** and **C**). In **B** the medial and lateral menisci (**18** and **22**) lie between the condyles of the femur and tibia (**4** and **9**, **7** and **12**), with the anterior cruciate ligament (**19**) passing backwards and laterally from the upper surface of the tibia to the medial surface of the lateral condyle of the femur. Compare the MR image in **C** with the dissection in **B**.

In **D** the joint has been opened up by cutting through the quadriceps muscle (**26**) and the patellar ligament (**30**), and turning laterally the large flap which includes the patella (**28**), in order to show the joint cavity from the front and the margins of the suprapatellar bursa (**27**) which is in direct continuity with the cavity of the knee joint.

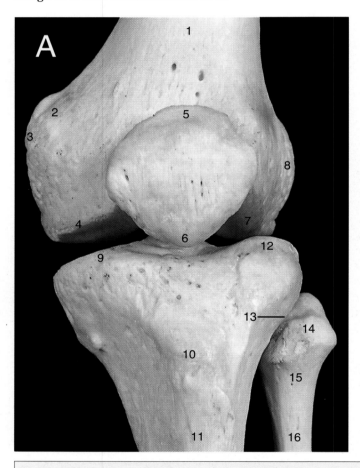

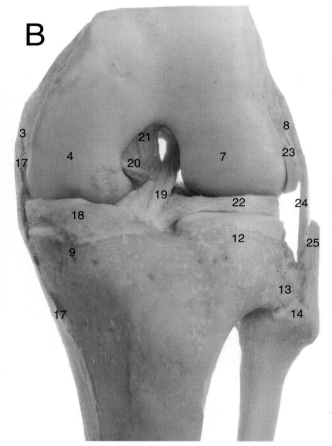

- The lateral ligament (**B24**, properly called the fibular collateral ligament) is a rounded cord about 5 cm long, passing from the lateral epicondyle of the femur (**B8**) to the head of the fibula (**B14**).

- The medial ligament (**B17**, properly called the tibial collateral ligament) is a broad flat band about 12 cm long passing from the medial epicondyle of the femur (**B3**) to the medial side of the medial condyle of the

tibia (**B9**) and to an extensive area of the medial surface below the condyle. At the side it fuses with the medial meniscus (**B18**; see also page 29, **B18** and **19**); the lateral ligament (**B24**) does not fuse with the lateral meniscus (**B22**), to which the tendon of popliteus has an attachment (page 29, **C28**).

- For notes on the cruciate ligaments and menisci see page 29

1	Shaft of femur	17	Medial ligament
2	Adductor tubercle	18	Medial meniscus
3	Medial epicondyle	19	Anterior cruciate ligament
4	Medial condyle	20	Anterior meniscofemoral ligament
5	Base of patella	21	Posterior cruciate ligament
6	Apex of patella	22	Lateral meniscus
7	Lateral condyle	23	Popliteus tendon
8	Lateral epicondyle	24	Lateral ligament
9	Medial condyle of tibia	25	Biceps tendon
10	Tibial tuberosity	26	Quadriceps femoris
11	Shaft	27	Margins of suprapatellar bursa
12	Lateral condyle	28	Posterior surface of patella
13	Superior tibiofibular joint (with capsule in **B**)	29	Infrapatellar fat pad
14	Head of fibula	30	Patellar ligament
15	Neck	31	Deep infrapatellar bursa
16	Shaft		

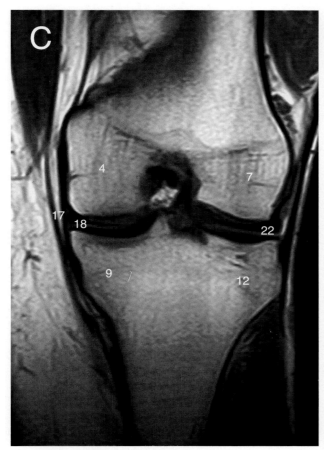

By courtesy of Dr Kate Stevens

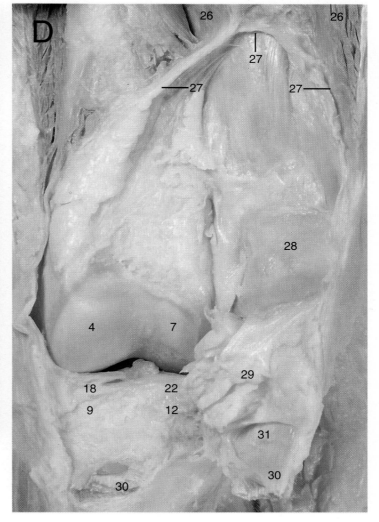

KNEE
Left knee joint
A Bones, from behind
B Ligaments, from behind
C Upper surface of tibia with ligaments, from above

The joint in **B** is partly flexed, showing less of the articular surfaces of the femoral condyles (**4** and **6**) than in **A**. In **B** the posterior cruciate ligament (**20**) spills over on to the uppermost part of the posterior surface of the tibia. The attachment of the medial meniscus (**19**) to the medial ligament (**18**) is clearly seen; the lateral meniscus (**23**) has no attachment to the lateral ligament (**24**) but gives rise to the posterior meniscofemoral ligament (**22**) which lies on the surface

of the posterior cruciate ligament (**20**), here obscuring the anterior meniscofemoral ligament (**27**).

The view in **C** demonstrates the shapes of the medial and lateral menisci (**19** and **23**), the tibial attachments of the anterior and posterior cruciate ligaments (**21** and **20**) and the anterior and posterior meniscofemoral ligaments (**27** and **22**) which pass respectively in front of and behind the posterior cruciate ligament (**20**).

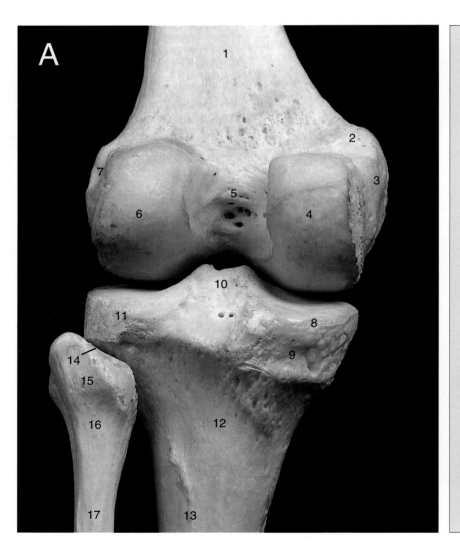

1 Popliteal surface of femur
2 Adductor tubercle
3 Medial epicondyle
4 Medial condyle
5 Intercondylar fossa
6 Lateral condyle
7 Lateral epicondyle
8 Medial condyle of tibia
9 Groove for semimembranosus insertion
10 Intercondylar eminence
11 Lateral condyle
12 Popliteal surface of tibia
13 Soleal line
14 Superior tibiofibular joint (with capsule in **B**)
15 Head of fibula
16 Neck
17 Shaft
18 Medial ligament
19 Medial meniscus
20 Posterior cruciate ligament
21 Anterior cruciate ligament
22 Posterior meniscofemoral ligament
23 Lateral meniscus (with marker under medial margin in **C**)
24 Lateral ligament
25 Popliteus tendon
26 Biceps tendon
27 Anterior meniscofemoral ligament
28 Attachment of popliteus to lateral meniscus

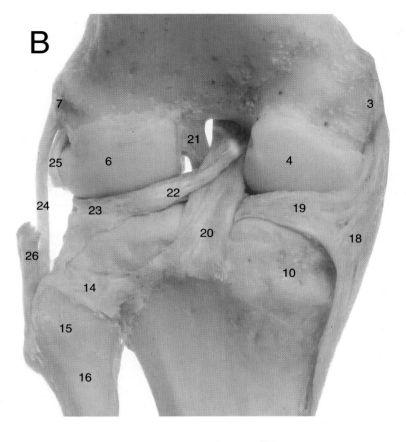

B

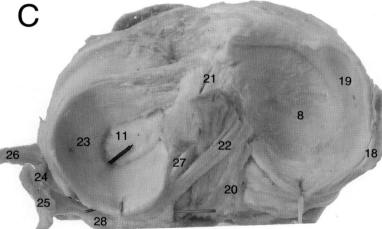

C

- The cruciate ligaments are named from their attachments to the tibia.

- The anterior cruciate ligament (**C21**), from the front of the upper surface of the tibia, passes upwards, backwards and laterally to become attached to the medial side of the lateral condyle of the femur (page 26, **B19**).

- The posterior cruciate ligament (**C20**), from the back of the upper surface and the very top of the posterior surface of the tibia, passes upwards, forwards and medially to become attached to lateral side of the medial condyle of the femur (page 26, **B21**).

- The anterior and posterior meniscofemoral ligaments (**C27** and **C22**) arise from the back of the lateral meniscus and run upwards and forwards like a two-pronged fork embracing the posterior cruciate ligament (**C20**) at its front and back and fusing with it.

- The C-shaped fibrocartilaginous menisci (**C19** and **C23**) are attached by their ends (the horns of the menisci) to the intercondylar area of the upper surface of the tibia.

- Muscles producing movements at the knee joint:
  Flexion (bending the leg backwards): semimembranosus, semitendinosus, biceps, gracilis, sartorius, gastrocnemius and popliteus.

  Extension (straightening the flexed knee): vastus medialis, vastus intermedius, vastus lateralis, rectus femoris, and tensor fasciae latae and gluteus maximus acting via the iliotibial tract.

  Medial rotation of the flexed leg (rotating the leg medially in the long axis of the leg): semimembranosus, semitendinosus, gracilis, sartorius and popliteus.

  Lateral rotation of the flexed leg (rotating the leg laterally in the long axis of the leg): biceps.

- Because of the shape of the articulating surfaces and the tension in the ligaments, there is some medial rotation of the femur on the tibia towards the end of extension (assuming the tibia to be fixed); this is the so-called 'locking of the knee joint'. To begin flexion, popliteus 'unlocks' the joint by causing some lateral rotation of the femur on the tibia (assuming the tibia to be fixed); the other flexors can then carry on the movement.

KNEE
Popliteal fossa and back of the knee
A Right popliteal fossa
B Surface landmarks of the flexed right knee, from the lateral side

In **A** the fascia that forms the roof of the fossa and the fat within it have been removed. At the upper part of the fossa, biceps (**10**) is on the lateral side with the common peroneal nerve (**9**) at its posterior border, and semi-membranosus (**3**) with semitendinosus (**4**) overlying it are on the medial side. At the lower part of the fossa, the medial head of gastrocnemius (**15**) is on the medial side, while on the lateral side plantaris (**11**) lies just above the lateral head of gastrocnemius (**12**). Of the principal structures within the fossa, the tibial nerve (**7**) is the most superficial, with the popliteal vein (**6**) behind it and the popliteal artery (**5**) deep to the vein.

In the lateral view in **B**, the ridge formed by the iliotibial tract (**18**) lies above (anterior to) the tendon of biceps (**10**), at the lateral boundary of the popliteal fossa (**25**). Below the head of the fibula (**24**) the common peroneal nerve (**9**) is palpable and can be rolled against the neck of the bone.

1	Sartorius
2	Gracilis
3	Semimembranosus
4	Semitendinosus
5	Popliteal artery
6	Popliteal vein
7	Tibial nerve
8	Lateral cutaneous nerve of calf
9	Common peroneal nerve
10	Biceps
11	Plantaris
12	Lateral head of gastrocnemius
13	Small saphenous vein (double)
14	Sural nerve
15	Medial head of gastrocnemius
16	Nerve to medial head ⎤ of
17	Nerve to lateral head ⎦ gastrocnemius
18	Iliotibial tract
19	Patella
20	Margin of lateral condyle of femur
21	Patellar ligament
22	Tuberosity of tibia
23	Margin of lateral condyle of tibia
24	Head of fibula
25	Popliteal fossa

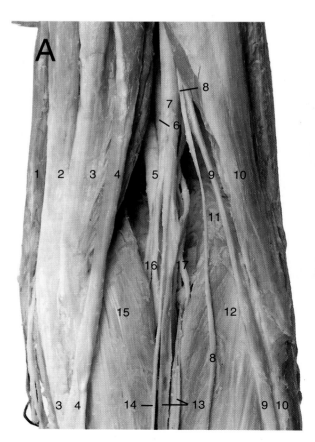

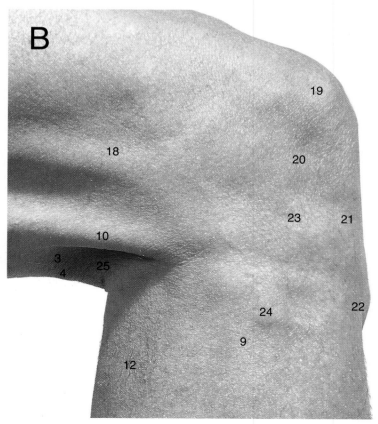

KNEE
Popliteal fossa and back of the knee
C Right popliteus muscle and knee joint capsule, from behind

Most of gastrocnemius, soleus and other muscles have been removed to display popliteus (**6**) and the posterior surface of the knee joint capsule (**13**), which is reinforced by the tendinous fibres of semimembranosus (**11**) that form the oblique popliteal ligament (**12**).

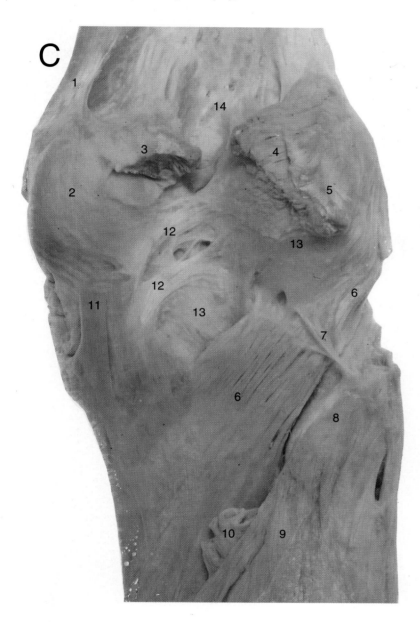

1	Adductor magnus
2	Capsule overlying medial condyle of femur
3	Medial head of gastrocnemius
4	Plantaris
5	Lateral head of gastrocnemius
6	Popliteus
7	Arcuate popliteal ligament
8	Head of fibula
9	Soleus
10	Popliteal vessels and tibial nerve
11	Semimembranosus
12	Oblique popliteal ligament
13	Capsule of knee joint
14	Popliteal surface of femur

- The deep position of the popliteal artery (**A5**) - deep to the popliteal vein (**A6**) which in turn is deep to the tibial nerve (**A7**) - makes feeling the popliteal pulse difficult. It is best felt from the front, grasping the sides of the knee with both hands, placing the thumbs beside the patella and pressing the tips of the fingers deeply into the midline of the fossa.

- The slender arcuate popliteal ligament (**C7**) arches over popliteus (**C6**) as it enters the joint capsule to reach the lateral side of the lateral condyle of the femur.

LEG AND FOOT SURVEY
Muscles and superficial vessels and nerves of the left leg and foot
A From the front
B From the medial side
C From the lateral side
D From behind
E From behind, with gastrocnemius detached
F From behind, with gastrocnemius, plantaris and soleus detached

Skin, subcutaneous tissue and most of the deep fascia have been removed, and different aspects of the same specimen are shown. Lateral to the medial (subcutaneous) surface (**A2**) and anterior border of the tibia is the largest muscle of the front of the leg, tibialis anterior (**A6, C6**), which becomes tendinous in the lower part of the leg and has the tendons of extensor hallucis longus (**A7**) and extensor digitorum longus (**A8**) lateral to it. On the medial side the bulk of gastrocnemius (**A3, B3**) and the underlying soleus (**A4**) overlie the flexor muscles whose tendons pass behind the medial malleolus (**B9**) – tibialis posterior (**B19**), flexor digitorum

longus (**B18**) and flexor hallucis longus (**B16**), in that order from front to back. On the lateral side, peroneus longus (**C23**) largely overlies peroneus brevis (**C25**); their tendons pass behind the lateral malleolus (**C10**). At the back gastrocnemius (**D3**) has been detached at its upper end to show the underlying soleus (**E4**), which in turn has been detached with plantaris (**E31**) in **F** to display the underlying flexor muscle — tibialis posterior (**F19**), the deepest muscle, which is overlapped by flexor hallucis longus (**F16**) on the lateral side and flexor digitorum longus (**F18**) on the medial side.

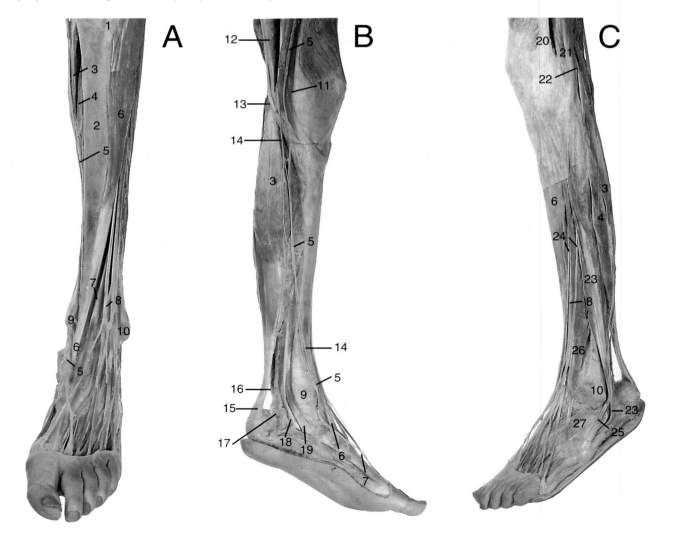

1 Patellar ligament (lower edge)	**18** Flexor digitorum longus
2 Medial surface of tibia	**19** Tibialis posterior
3 Gastrocnemius	**20** Iliotibial tract
4 Soleus	**21** Biceps femoris
5 Great saphenous vein	**22** Common peroneal nerve
6 Tibialis anterior	**23** Peroneus longus
7 Extensor hallucis longus	**24** Superficial peroneal nerve
8 Extensor digitorum longus	**25** Peroneus brevis
9 Medial malleolus	**26** Peroneus tertius
10 Lateral malleolus	**27** Extensor digitorum brevis
11 Sartorius	**28** Semimembranosus
12 Gracilis	**29** Small saphenous vein
13 Semitendinosus	**30** Sural nerve
14 Saphenous nerve	**31** Plantaris
15 Tendo calcaneus	**32** Tibial nerve
16 Flexor hallucis longus	**33** Popliteal vein overlying artery
17 Tibial nerve and posterior tibial vessels	**34** Fascia over popliteus

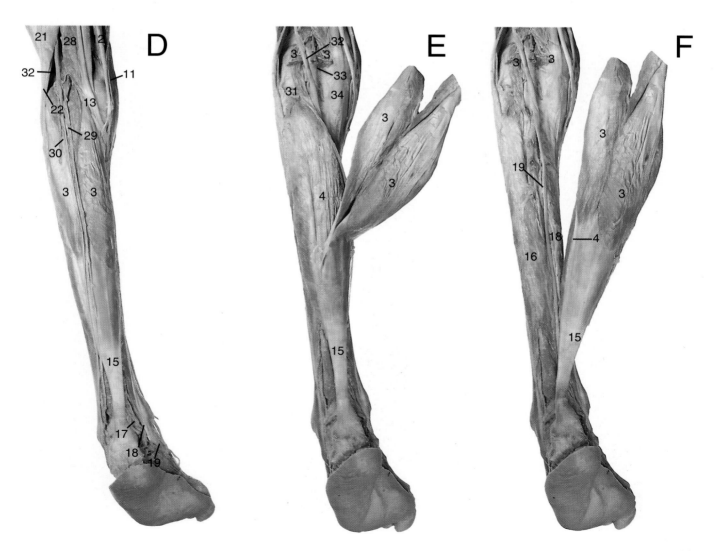

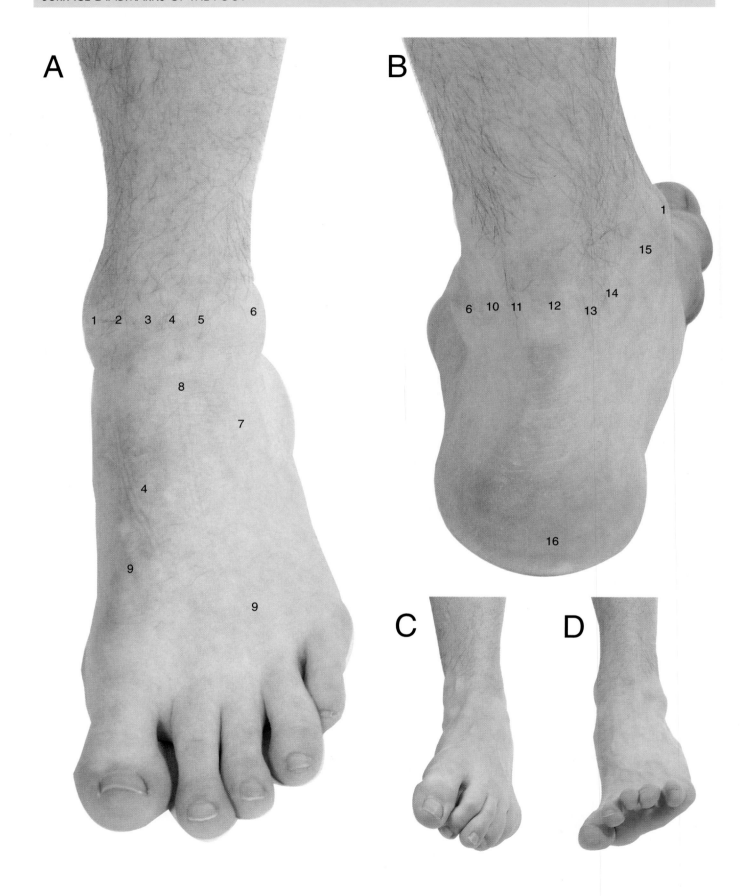

SURFACE LANDMARKS OF THE FOOT
Surface landmarks of the left foot
A From the front (dorsal surface, dorsum)
B From behind
C From the front, in inversion
D From the front, in eversion with abduction of toes
E From below (plantar surface, sole)
F Imprint of sole when weight-bearing (viewed through a glass plate)

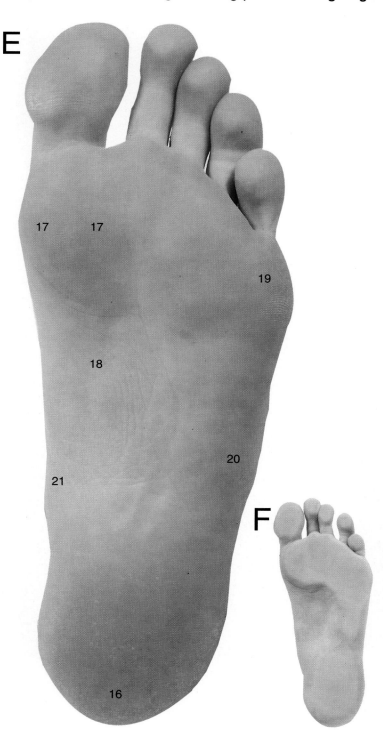

1 Medial malleolus
2 Great saphenous vein and saphenous nerve
3 Tibialis anterior
4 Extensor hallucis longus
5 Extensor digitorum longus
6 Lateral malleolus
7 Extensor digitorum brevis
8 Dorsalis pedis artery
9 Dorsal venous arch
10 Peroneus longus and brevis
11 Small saphenous vein and sural nerve
12 Tendo calcaneus
13 Flexor hallucis longus
14 Posterior tibial artery and tibial nerve
15 Flexor digitorum longus and tibialis posterior
16 Tuberosity of calcaneus
17 Sesamoid bones under head of first metatarsal
18 Base of first metatarsal
19 Head of fifth metatarsal
20 Tuberosity of base of fifth metatarsal
21 Tuberosity of navicular

- **Definition of movements**

Extension: from the Latin for straightening out, but as far as the ankle and foot are concerned it means bending the foot and/or toes upwards, and is also known as dorsiflexion.

Flexion: from the Latin for bending. In the ankle and foot it means bending the foot and/or toes downwards, which is also known as plantarflexion.

Abduction: from the Latin for moving away. In the foot it means spreading the toes apart (the corresponding movement of the fingers is much more extensive).

Adduction: from the Latin for moving towards. In the foot it means drawing the toes together.

Inversion: from the Latin for turning in – turning the foot so that the sole faces more inwards (medially).

Eversion: from the Latin for turning out – moving the foot so that the sole faces more outwards (laterally) (a more limited movement than inversion).

For further details see pages 81 and 93.

SURFACE LANDMARKS OF THE FOOT

Surface landmarks of the left foot
A From the medial side
B In dorsiflexion (extension)
C In plantarflexion (flexion)
D From the lateral side

1 Tendo calcaneus
2 Flexor hallucis longus
3 Posterior tibial artery and tibial nerve
4 Flexor digitorum longus and tibialis posterior
5 Medial malleolus
6 Great saphenous vein and saphenous nerve
7 Tibialis anterior
8 Extensor hallucis longus
9 Head of first metatarsal
10 Sesamoid bone
11 Tuberosity of navicular
12 Sustentaculum tali
13 Tuberosity of calcaneus
14 Small saphenous vein and sural nerve
15 Peroneus longus and brevis
16 Lateral malleolus
17 Extensor digitorum brevis
18 Extensor digitorum longus
19 Tuberosity of base of fifth metatarsal
20 Head of fifth metatarsal

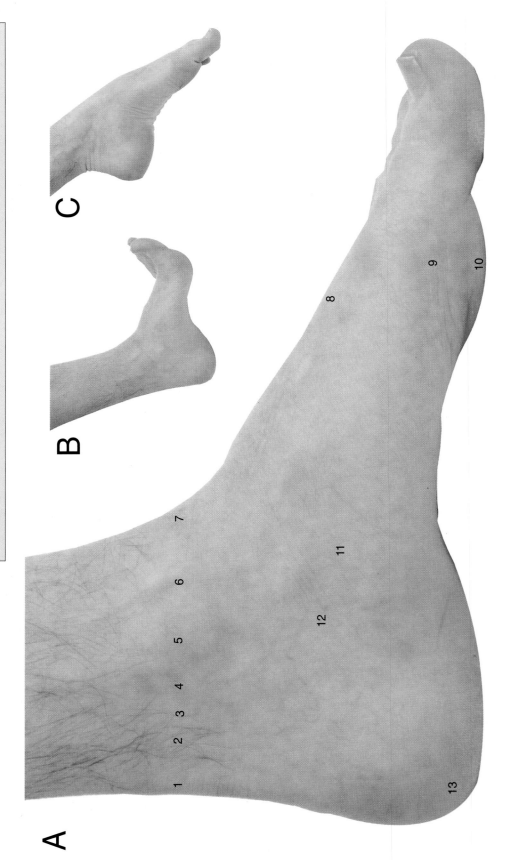

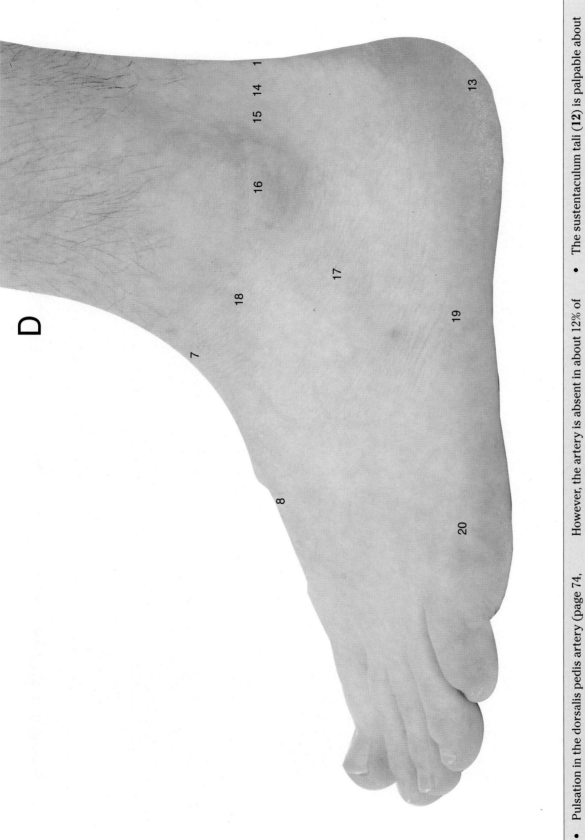

D

- Pulsation in the dorsalis pedis artery (page 74, **14**) is normally palpable between the tendons of extensor hallucis longus (**8**) and extensor digitorum longus (**18**), on a line from the midpoint between the medial and lateral malleoli to the proximal end of the first intermetatarsal space.

However, the artery is absent in about 12% of feet (see page 75).

- Pulsation in the posterior tibial artery (**3**) is normally palpable behind the medial malleolus (**5**), 2.5 cm in front of the medial border of the tendo calcaneus.

- The sustentaculum tali (**12**) is palpable about 2.5 cm below the tip of the medial malleolus (**5**).

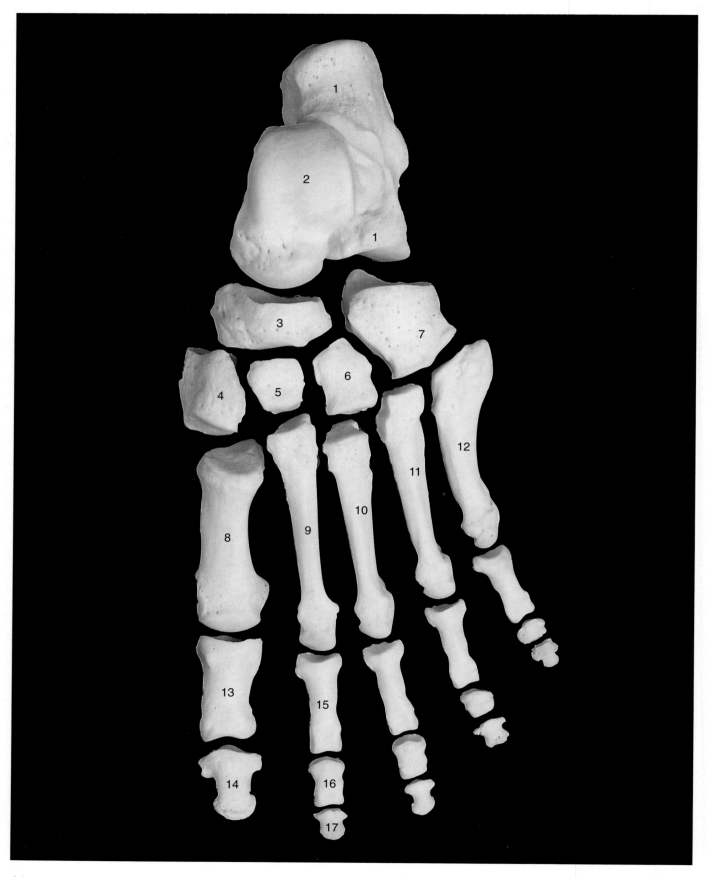

SKELETON OF THE FOOT
Bones of the left foot, from above

The talus and calcaneus remain articulated with each other but the remainder have been disarticulated

1	Calcaneus
2	Talus
3	Navicular
4	Medial cuneiform
5	Intermediate cuneiform
6	Lateral cuneiform
7	Cuboid
8	First metatarsal
9	Second metatarsal
10	Third metatarsal
11	Fourth metatarsal
12	Fifth metatarsal
13	Proximal phalanx of great toe
14	Distal phalanx of great toe
15	Proximal phalanx of second toe
16	Middle phalanx of second toe
17	Distal phalanx of second toe

- **Bones of the tarsus**
  Talus
  Calcaneus
  Navicular bone
  Cuboid bone
  Medial, intermediate and lateral cuneiform bones

- **Bones of the metatarsus**
  First to fifth metatarsal bones, numbered from medial to lateral

- **Bones of the toes or digits**
  Phalanges – a proximal and a distal phalanx for the great toe; proximal, middle and distal phalanges for each of the second to fifth toes

- The **hindfoot** consists of the talus and calcaneus.

- The **midfoot** consists of the navicular, cuboid and cuneiform bones.

- The **forefoot** consists of the metatarsal bones and phalanges.

- **Sesamoid bones** – two always present in the tendons of flexor hallucis brevis. For others see page 41.

- **Origin and meaning of some names associated with the foot** (some older names for bones are given in brackets)

Tibia:	Latin for a flute or pipe; when held upside down, the shin bone has a fanciful resemblance to this wind instrument.
Fibula:	Latin for a pin or skewer; the long thin bone of the leg. Adjective fibular or peroneal, which is from the Greek for pin (see the last note on page 11).
Tarsus:	Greek for a wicker frame, in the basic framework for the back of the foot.
Metatarsus:	Greek for beyond the tarsus; the forepart of the foot.
Talus: (astragalus)	Latin (Greek) for one of a set of dice; viewed from above the main part of the talus has a rather square appearance.
Calcaneus: (os calcis, calcaneum)	From the Greek for heel; the heel bone.
Navicular. (scaphoid)	Latin (Greek) for boat-shaped; the navicular bone roughly resembles a saucer-shaped coracle.
Cuboid:	Greek for cube-shaped.
Cuneiform:	Latin for wedge-shaped.
Phalanx:	Greek for a row of soldiers; a row of bones in the toes. Plural phalanges.
Sesamoid:	Greek for shaped like a sesame seed.
Digitus:	Latin for finger or toe. Digiti and digitorum are the genitive singular and genitive plural – of the toe(s).
Hallux:	Latin for the great toe. Hallucis is the genitive singular – of the great toe.
Dorsum:	Latin for back; the upper surface of the foot. Adjective dorsal.
Plantar:	adjective from planta, Latin for the sole of the foot.

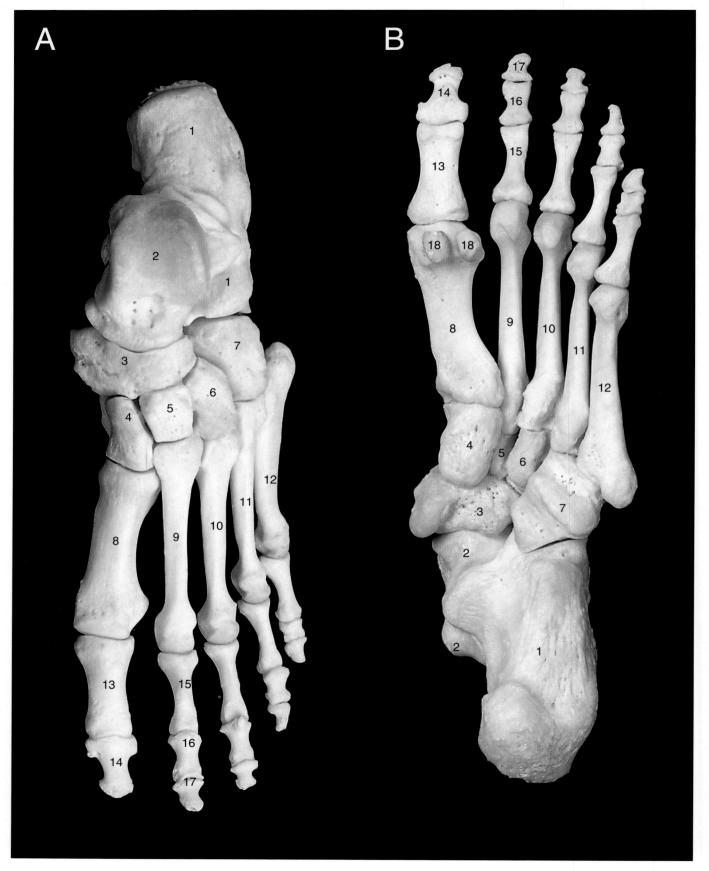

SKELETON OF THE FOOT
Articulated bones of the left foot
A From above (dorsal surface)
B From below (plantar surface)

1	Calcaneus	10	Third metatarsal
2	Talus	11	Fourth metatarsal
3	Navicular	12	Fifth metatarsal
4	Medial cuneiform	13	Proximal phalanx of great toe
5	Intermediate cuneiform	14	Distal phalanx of great toe
6	Lateral cuneiform	15	Proximal phalanx of second toe
7	Cuboid	16	Middle phalanx of second toe
8	First metatarsal	17	Distal phalanx of second toe
9	Second metatarsal	18	Sesamoid bones

- **Sesamoid bones**
  One in each of the two tendons of flexor hallucis brevis, articulating with the plantar surface of the head of the first metatarsal (**B18**).
  Others may be present in similar positions in flexor tendons under other metatarsophalangeal or interphalangeal joints, or in other tendons, especially those of tibialis anterior and peroneus longus (page 100, **B14**)

- During the preparation of dried bones, the hyaline cartilage on articulating surfaces is lost, so that when rearticulating bones an exact fit is not possible. The thickness of the cartilage on joint surface is best appreciated in sections of bones, as on pages 20 and 86–97

- The talus (**2**) is the uppermost foot bone, forming the ankle joint with the tibia and fibula. For details see pages 48-57.

- The calcaneus (**1**) is the most posterior and the largest foot bone, forming the heel. For details see pages 58-59.

- The navicular bone (**3**) lies in front of the talus, on the medial side of the foot. For details see page 60.

- The cuboid bone (**7**) lies in front of the calcaneus, on the lateral side of the foot. For details see page 60.

- The three cuneiform bones - medial, intermediate and lateral (**4**, **5** and **6**) - lie in front of the navicular bone. For details see page 61.

- The first, second and third metatarsal bones (**8**, **9** and **10**) are in front of the three cuneiforms, and the fourth and fifth metatarsal bones (**11** and **12**) are in front of the cuboid bone. For details see pages 62-63.

- The phalanges (**13-17**) are the bones of the toes. Each proximal phalanx articulates with the head of a metatarsal bone. Each phalanx has a base (at the proximal end), body, and head (at the distal end). The body is convex on the dorsal (upper) surface, and concave on the plantar surface. See pages 38-47.

- Very occasionally some accessory bones may be present in the foot. The commonest is the os trigonum, formed by the lateral tubercle of the posterior process of the talus; others may be formed by the tuberosity of the navicular and the tuberosity of the base of the fifth metatarsal. They must not be confused with fractures of the normal bones.

- **Ossification of foot bones**
  All the tarsal bones are ossified from one primary centre: calcaneus at the third fetal month, talus at the sixth fetal month, cuboid just before or just after birth, lateral cuneiform at 1 year, medial cuneiform at 2 years, intermediate cuneiform and navicular at 3 years.
  The calcaneus is the only tarsal bone to have a secondary centre: a thin plate of bone on the posterior surface, appearing at about 7 years and fusing during puberty.
  The metatarsal bones and phalanges have primary centres for their shafts at the second to fourth fetal months, and one secondary centre: at the base of the first metatarsal and bases of all the phalanges, but at the heads of the other metatarsals. These begin to ossify at 2 to 6 years and fuse at about 18 years.
  All dates given are subject to considerable variation, and ossification tends to occur earlier in females.

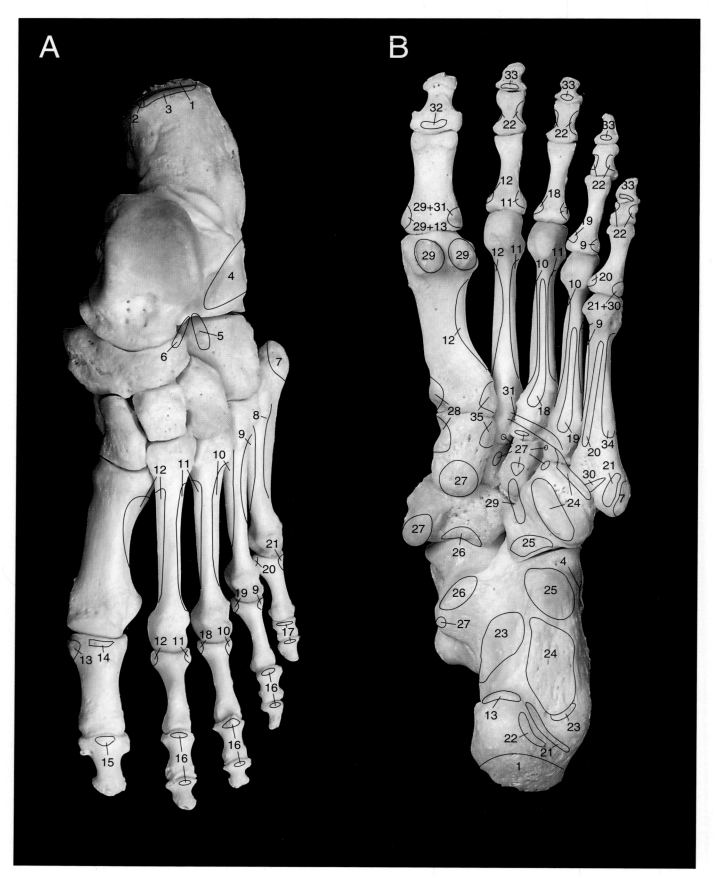

SKELETON OF THE FOOT
Attachments of muscles and major ligaments to the bones of the left foot
A From above (dorsal surface)
B From below (plantar surface)

1 Tendo calcaneus
2 Plantaris
3 Area for bursa
4 Extensor digitorum brevis
5 Calcaneocuboid part ⎤
6 Calcaneonavicular part ⎦ of bifurcate ligament
7 Peroneus brevis
8 Peroneus tertius
9 Fourth ⎤
10 Third ⎥
11 Second ⎥ dorsal interosseus
12 First ⎦
13 Abductor hallucis
14 Extensor hallucis brevis
15 Extensor hallucis longus
16 Extensor digitorum longus and brevis
17 Extensor digitorum longus

18 First ⎤
19 Second ⎥ plantar interosseus
20 Third ⎦
21 Abductor digiti minimi
22 Flexor digitorum brevis
23 Flexor accessorius
24 Long plantar ligament
25 Plantar calcaneocuboid (short plantar) ligament
26 Plantar calcaneonavicular (spring) ligament
27 Tibialis posterior
28 Tibialis anterior
29 Flexor hallucis brevis
30 Flexor digiti minimi brevis
31 Adductor hallucis
32 Flexor hallucis longus
33 Flexor digitorum longus
34 Opponens digiti minimi (occasional part of **30**)
35 Peroneus longus

- Flexor accessorius is alternatively known as quadratus plantae.

SKELETON OF THE FOOT
Articulated bones of the left foot
A From the medial side
B From the lateral side

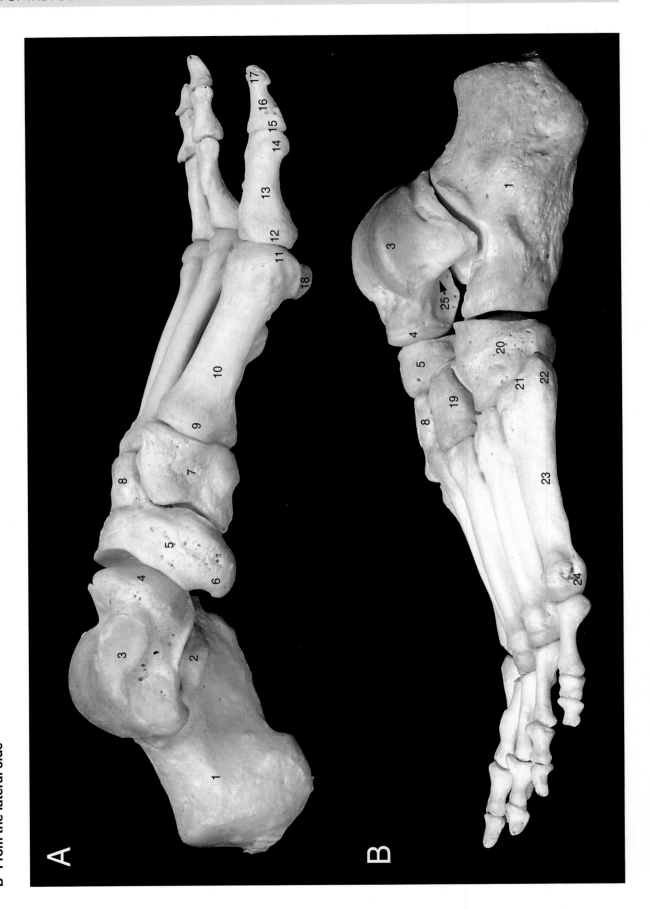

- When standing (as can be seen from the imprint of a wet foot on the floor or when viewed through a glass plate – see page 35, **F**) the parts of the foot in contact with the ground are the heel, the lateral margin of the foot, the pads under the metatarsal heads and the pads under the distal part of the toes.

- The medial margin of the foot is not normally in contact with the ground because of the height of the medial longitudinal arch (see pages 46 and 47). In flat foot the medial arch is lower with an increasingly large imprint on the medial side.

- The body weight when standing is borne by the tuberosity of the calcaneus and the heads of the metatarsals, especially the first (with the sesamoid bones underneath it) and the fifth. As

the foot bends forwards in walking the other metatarsal heads take increasingly more of the load. With further raising of the heel the toe pads become pressed to the ground and so take some of the weight off the metatarsals.

- Although the forearm and hand have many muscles that are similar in name and action to those of the leg and foot, their normal use in everyday life is different.
  In the upper limb the muscles work from above to produce intricate movements of the thumb and fingers in a free limb.
  In the lower limb the toes have to be stabilized on the ground so that muscles can work from below to produce the propulsive movements of walking.

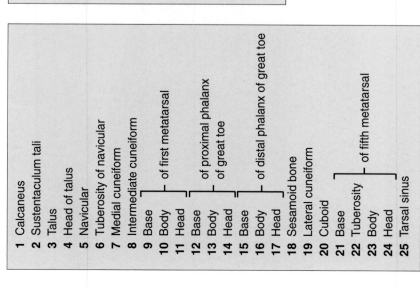

1 Calcaneus
2 Sustentaculum tali
3 Talus
4 Head of talus
5 Navicular
6 Tuberosity of navicular
7 Medial cuneiform
8 Intermediate cuneiform
9 Base
10 Body ⎱ of first metatarsal
11 Head
12 Base
13 Body ⎱ of proximal phalanx
14 Head ⎰ of great toe
15 Base
16 Body ⎱ of distal phalanx of great toe
17 Head
18 Sesamoid bone
19 Lateral cuneiform
20 Cuboid
21 Base
22 Tuberosity ⎱ of fifth metatarsal
23 Body ⎰
24 Head
25 Tarsal sinus

SKELETON OF THE FOOT
Bones of the left longitudinal arches, transverse tarsal joint, and other joints

A Bones of the medial longitudinal arch, from above
B Bones of the lateral longitudinal arch, from the lateral side
C The transverse tarsal joint, disarticulated, from above

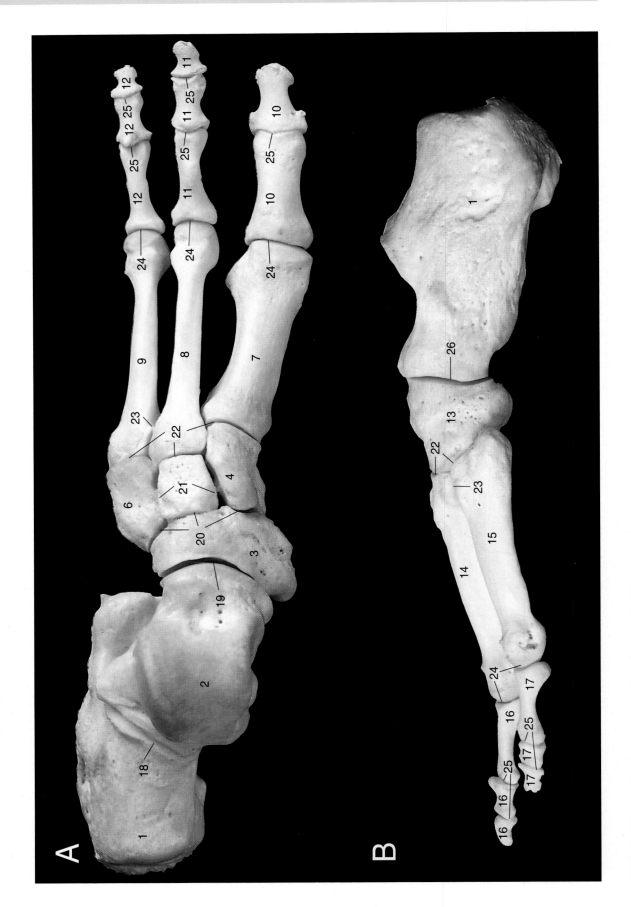

- The bones of the medial longitudinal arch (**A**) are the calcaneus, talus, navicular, the three cuneiforms and the medial three metatarsal bones.

- The bones of the lateral longitudinal arch (**B**) are the calcaneus, cuboid and the two lateral metatarsal bones.

- The transverse arch is formed by the cuboid and cuneiform bones and the adjacent parts of the five metatarsals (those of each foot forming one half of the whole arch). At the level of the metatarsal heads the arched form is no longer present.

- The medial longitudinal arch is higher than the lateral.

- While the shape of the individual bones determines the shapes of the arches, the *maintenance* of the arches in the *stationary* foot (standing in the normal upright position) depends largely on the ligaments in the sole (where they are larger and stronger than those on the dorsum). As soon as movement occurs the long tendons and small muscles of the sole assume importance in maintaining the curved forms.

- The many joints of the foot contribute to its function as a *flexible* lever, and the word arch suggests an architectural rigidity that does not exist.

- On the medial side the plantar calcaneonavicular ligament (spring ligament) is of particular importance in supporting the head of the talus, and other structures that help to maintain the medial arch include the plantar aponeurosis, flexor hallucis longus, tibialis anterior and posterior, and the medial parts of flexor digitorum longus and brevis.

- The transverse tarsal joint (midtarsal joint) is the collective name for two joints – the calcaneocuboid joint, and the talonavicular part of the talocalcaneonavicular joint.

1 Calcaneus
2 Talus
3 Navicular
4 Medial cuneiform
5 Intermediate cuneiform
6 Lateral cuneiform
7 First metatarsal
8 Second metatarsal
9 Third metatarsal
10 Phalanges of great toe
11 Phalanges of second toe
12 Phalanges of third toe
13 Cuboid
14 Fourth metatarsal
15 Fifth metatarsal
16 Phalanges of fourth toe
17 Phalanges of fifth toe
18 Talocalcanean joint
19 Talonavicular part of talocalcaneonavicular joint
20 Cuneonavicular joint
21 Intercuneiform joints
22 Tarsometatarsal joints (cuneometatarsal and cuboideometatarsal)
23 Intermetatarsal joints
24 Metatarsophalangeal joints
25 Interphalangeal joints
26 Calcaneocuboid joint
27 Cuboideonavicular joint
28 Cuneocuboid joint

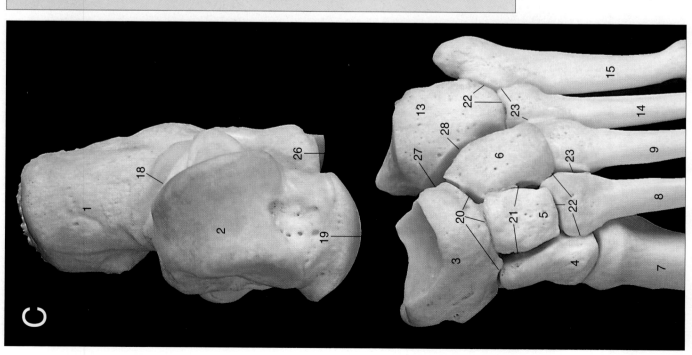

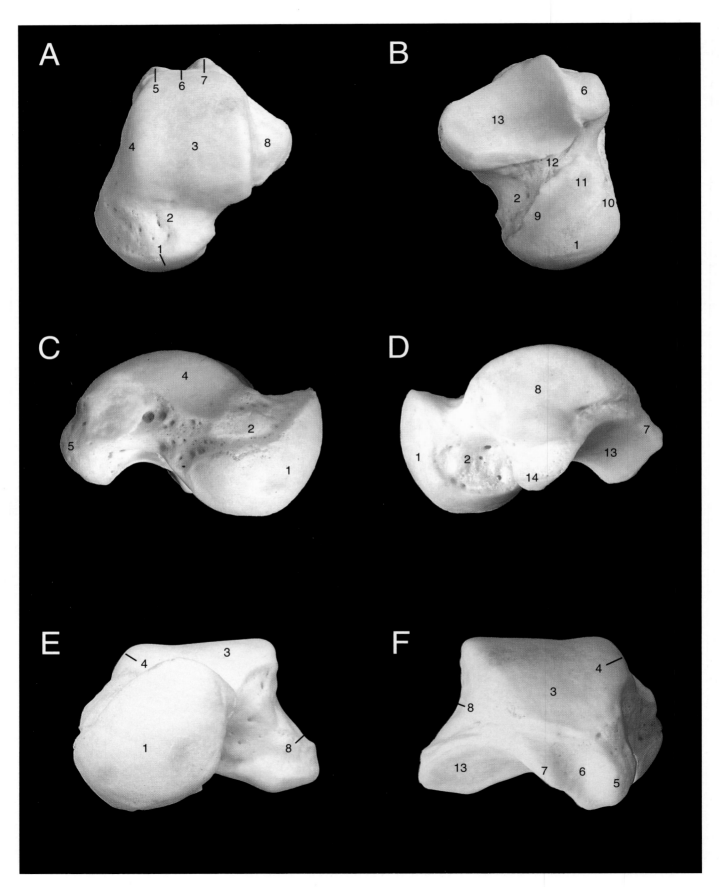

FOOT BONES
Left talus
A **From above**
B **From below**
C **From the medial side**
D **From the lateral side**
E **From the front**
F **From behind**

1 Head with articular surface for navicular
2 Neck
3 Trochlear surface of body, for inferior surface of tibia
4 Surface for medial malleolus
5 Medial tubercle ⎤
6 Groove for flexor hallucis longus tendon ⎬ of posterior process
7 Lateral tubercle ⎦
8 Surface for lateral malleolus
9 Anterior calcanean articular surface
10 Surface for plantar calcaneonavicular (spring) ligament
11 Middle calcanean articular surface
12 Sulcus tali
13 Posterior calcanean articular surface
14 Lateral process

Talus
- The uppermost foot bone, forming the ankle joint with the tibia and fibula.

- Formerly known as the astragalus.

- Articular facets on the upper surface and sides for the tibia and fibula, on the under surface for the calcaneus, and on the anterior surface (head) for the navicular.

- Unique among the foot bones in having no muscles attached to it.

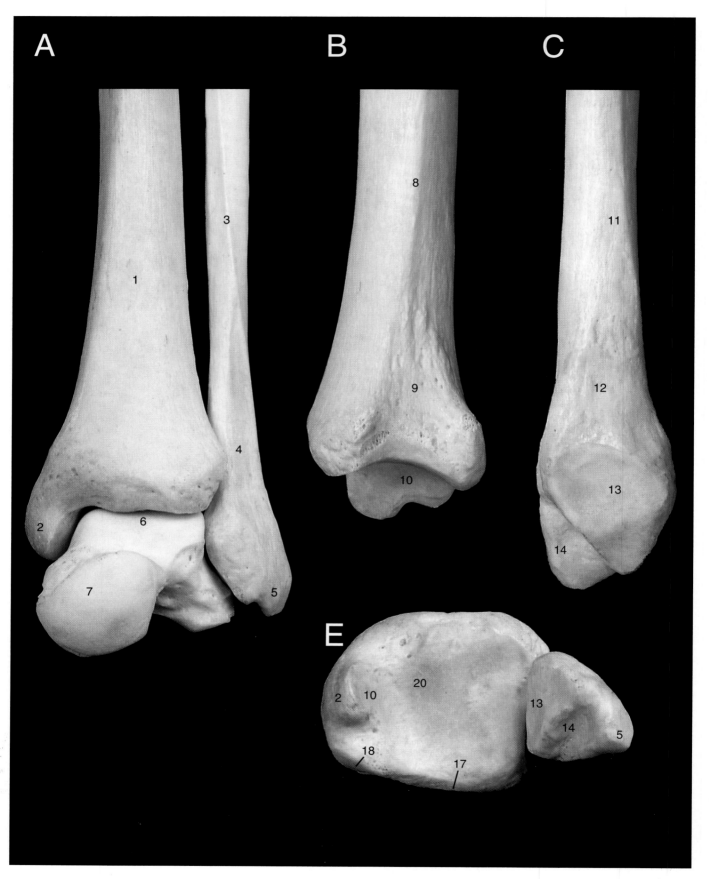

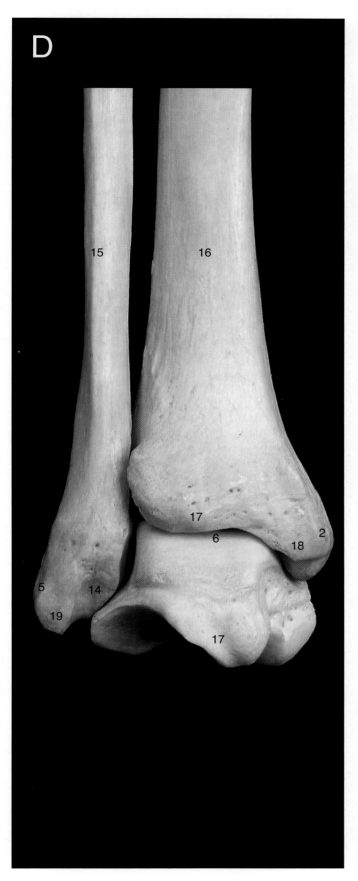

FOOT BONES

Left talus and the lower ends of the tibia and fibula

A **The talus, tibia and fibula, articulated, from the front**
B **The tibia from the lateral side**
C **The fibula from the medial side**
D **The talus, tibia and fibula, articulated, from behind**
E **The tibia and fibula, articulated, from below**

 1 Anterior surface ⎤
 2 Medial malleolus ⎦ of tibia
 3 Anterior border ⎤
 4 Triangular subcutaneous area ⎬ of fibula
 5 Lateral malleolus ⎦
 6 Trochlear surface of body ⎤ of talus
 7 Head ⎦
 8 Interosseous border ⎤
 9 Fibular notch ⎬ of tibia
10 Articular (lateral) surface of medial malleolus ⎦
11 Interosseous border ⎤
12 Surface for interosseous tibiofibular ligament ⎪
13 Articular (medial) surface of lateral malleolus ⎬ of fibula
14 Malleolar fossa ⎪
15 Posterior border ⎦
16 Posterior surface of tibia
17 Groove for flexor hallucis longus tendon
18 Groove for tibialis posterior tendon
19 Groove for peroneus brevis tendon
20 Inferior surface of tibia

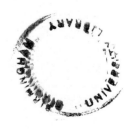

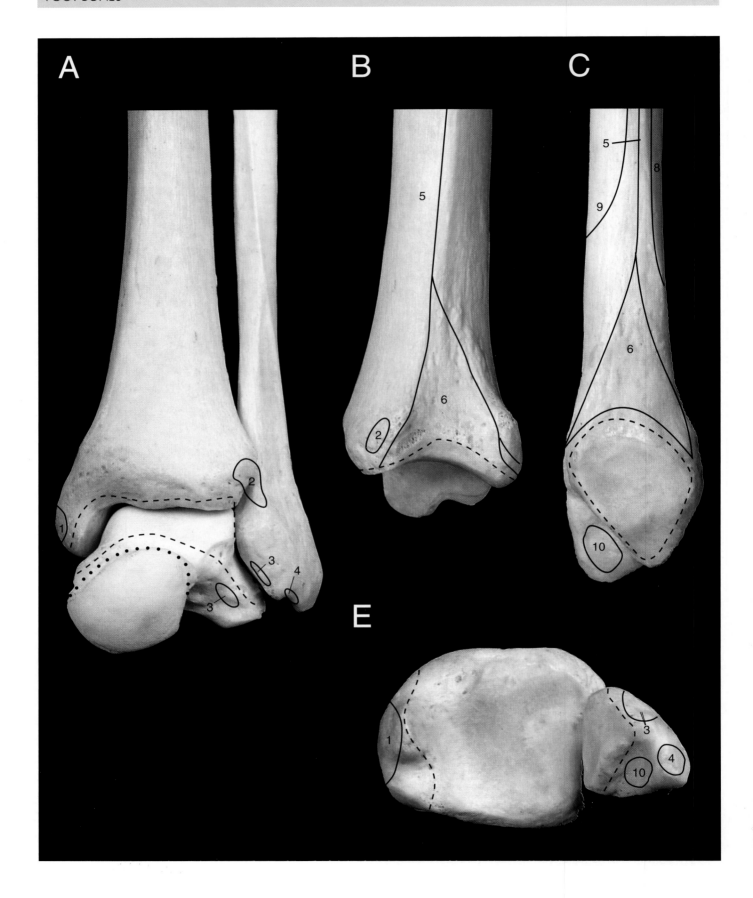

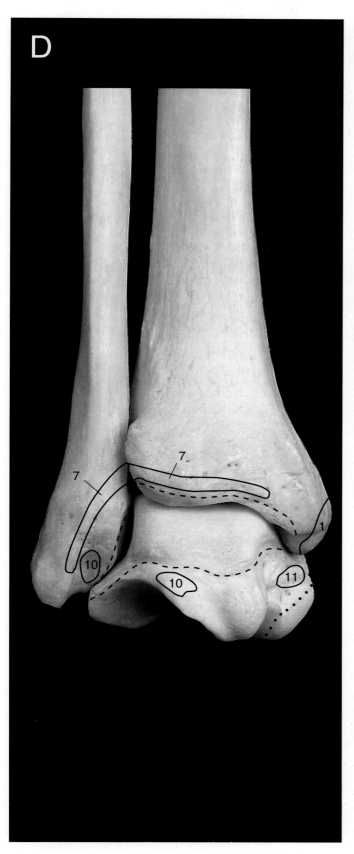

FOOT BONES
Left talus and the lower ends of the tibia and fibula, with ligamentous attachments in the ankle region

A The talus, tibia and fibula, articulated, from the front

B The tibia from the lateral side

C The fibula from the medial side

D The talus, tibia and fibula, articulated, from behind

E The tibia and fibula, articulated, from below

The attachment of the capsule of the ankle joint is indicated by the interrupted line, and that of the talo-calcaneonavicular joint by the dotted line.

1	Medial (deltoid) ligament
2	Anterior tibiofibular ligament
3	Anterior talofibular ligament
4	Calcaneofibular ligament
5	Interroseous membrane
6	Interosseous tibiofibular ligament
7	Posterior tibiofibular ligament
8	Peroneus tertius
9	Flexor hallucis longus
10	Posterior talofibular ligament
11	Deep part of medial (deltoid) ligament

- The interosseous tibiofibular ligament (**B** and **C,6**) is the main bond of union of the inferior tibiofibular joint.

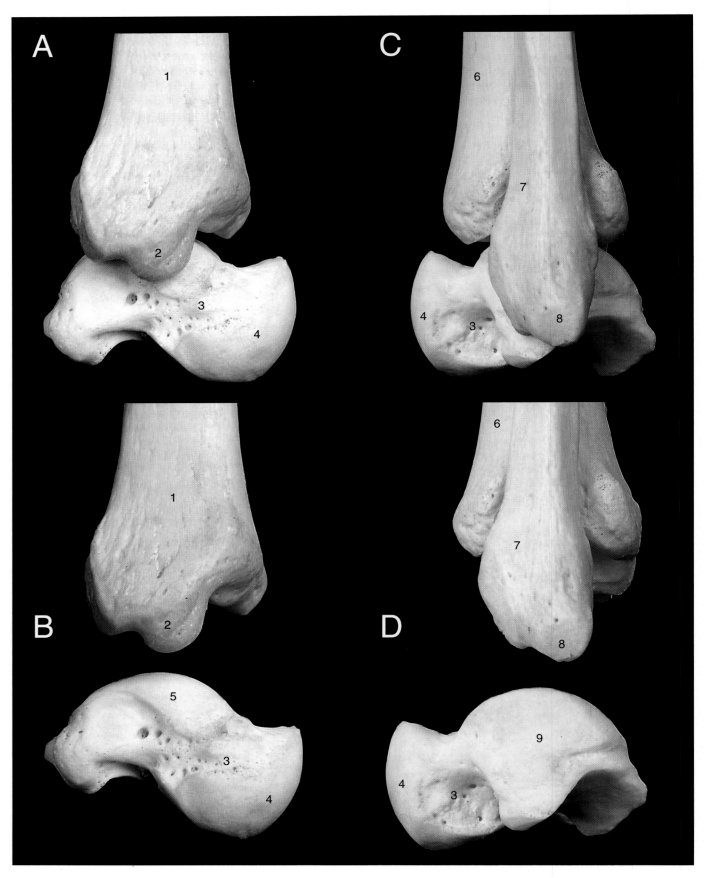

FOOT BONES

Left talus and the lower ends of the tibia and fibula
A The talus and tibia, articulated, from the medial side
B The talus and tibia, disarticulated, from the medial side
C The talus, tibia and fibula, articulated, from the lateral side
D The talus disarticulated from the tibia and fibula, from the lateral side

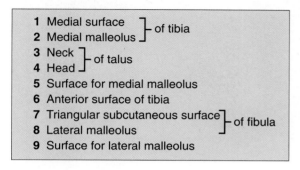

1 Medial surface ⎤ of tibia
2 Medial malleolus ⎦
3 Neck ⎤ of talus
4 Head ⎦
5 Surface for medial malleolus
6 Anterior surface of tibia
7 Triangular subcutaneous surface ⎤ of fibula
8 Lateral malleolus ⎦
9 Surface for lateral malleolus

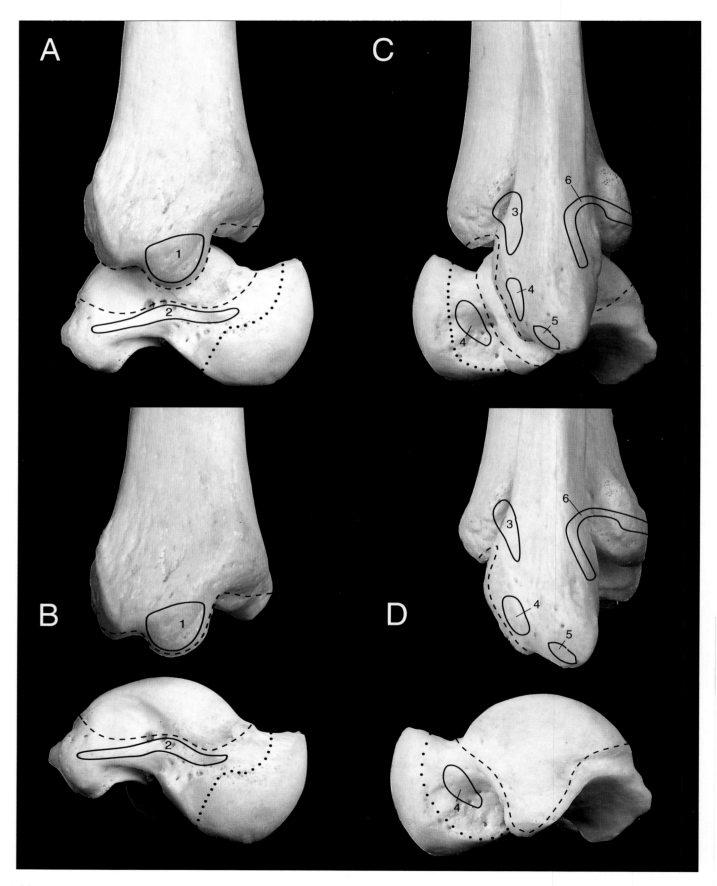

FOOT BONES

Left talus and the lower ends of the tibia and fibula, with ligamentous attachments in the ankle region
A The talus and tibia, articulated, from the medial side
B The talus and tibia, disarticulated, from the medial side
C The talus, tibia and fibula, articulated, from the lateral side
D The talus disarticulated from the tibia and fibula, from the lateral side

The attachment of the capsule of the ankle joint is indicated by the interrupted line, and that of the talo-calcaneonavicular joint by the dotted line.

1 Medial (deltoid) ligament
2 Deep part of medial (deltoid) ligament
3 Anterior tibiofibular ligament
4 Anterior talofibular ligament
5 Calcaneofibular ligament
6 Posterior tibiofibular ligament

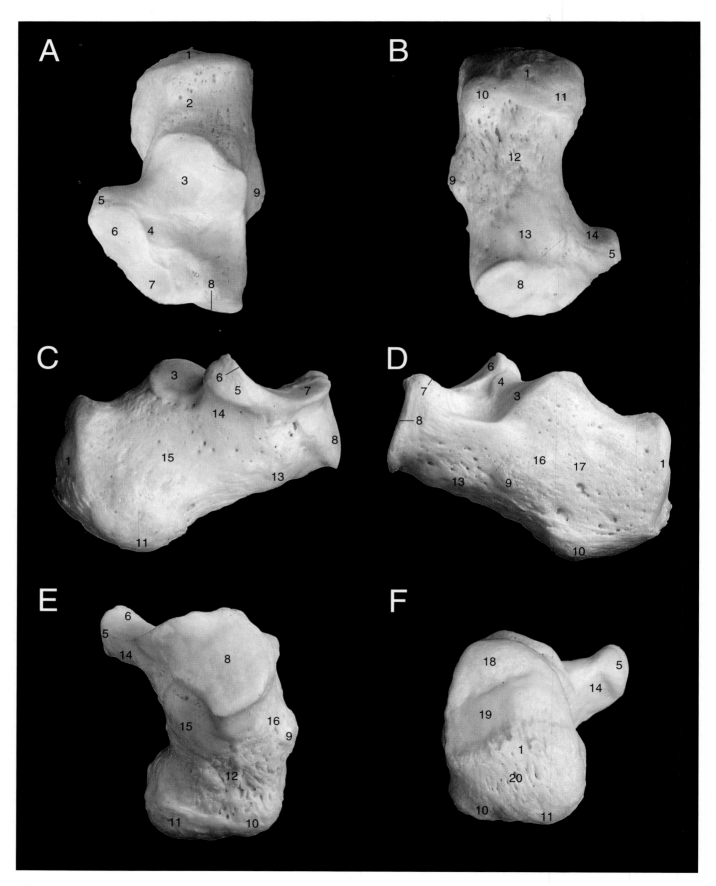

FOOT BONES

Left calcaneus

A From above
B From below
C From the medial side
D From the lateral side
E From the front
F From behind
G Articulated with the talus, from above
H With the talus disarticulated and turned upside down, with attachments

(Capsule of talocalcanean joint: interrupted line. Capsule of talocalcanean part of talocalcaneonavicular joint: dotted line)

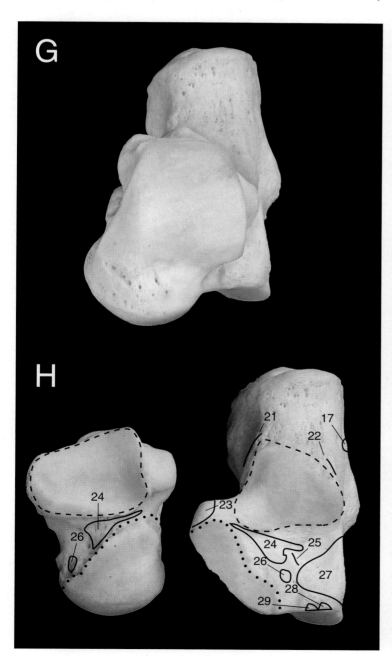

1	Posterior surface
2	Dorsal surface
3	Posterior articular surface for talus
4	Sulcus calcanei
5	Sustentaculun tali
6	Middle articular surface for talus
7	Anterior articular surface for talus
8	Articular surface for cuboid
9	Peroneal trochlea
10	Lateral process ⎤
11	Medial process ⎦ of tuberosity
12	Plantar surface
13	Anterior tubercle
14	Groove for flexor hallucis longus tendon
15	Medial surface
16	Lateral surface
17	Tubercle for calcaneofibular ligament
18	Surface for bursa
19	Surface for tendo calcaneus
20	Surface for fibrofatty tissue
21	Medial ⎤
22	Lateral ⎦ talocalcanean ligament
23	Tibiocalcanean part of medial (deltoid) ligament
24	Interosseous talocalcanean ligament
25	Inferior extensor retinaculum
26	Cervical ligament
27	Extensor digitorum brevis
28	Calcaneocuboid part
29	Calcaneonavicular part of bifurcate ligament

Calcaneus

- The largest foot bone, forming the heel.

- Formerly known as the calcaneum or os calcis.

- Articular facets on the upper surface for the talus and on the anterior surface for the cuboid.

- Prominent sustentaculum tali projecting medially.

- When the talus and calcaneus are articulated the sulcus tali (see page 48, **B12**) and sulcus calcanei (**4**) form the tarsal sinus (sinus tarsi).

FOOT BONES

Left navicular bone
A From above
B From below
C Proximal aspect
D Distal aspect

Left cuboid bone
E From above
F From below
G From the medial side
H From the lateral side
J Proximal aspect
K Distal aspect

1 Dorsal surface
2 Proximal surface for talus
3 Distal surface for cuneiforms
4 Plantar surface
5 Tuberosity
6 Facet for medial cuneiform ⎤
7 Facet for intermediate cuneiform ⎬ on distal surface
8 Facet for lateral cuneiform ⎦

9 Dorsal surface
10 Medial surface
11 Proximal surface for calcaneus
12 Lateral surface
13 Distal surface
14 Plantar surface
15 Groove for peroneus longus tendon
16 Tuberosity
17 Surface for lateral cuneiform
18 Surface for navicular
19 Facet for sesamoid bone in peroneus longus tendon
20 Facet for fifth metatarsal ⎤ on distal surface
21 Facet for fourth metatarsal ⎦

Navicular bone
• Formerly known as the scaphoid bone.

• Posterior articular facet for the talus; anterior articular facet for the three cuneiforms.

Cuboid bone
• Posterior articular facet for the calcaneus; anterior articular facet for the fourth and fifth metatarsals.

• Groove on the under surface for the tendon of peroneus longus.

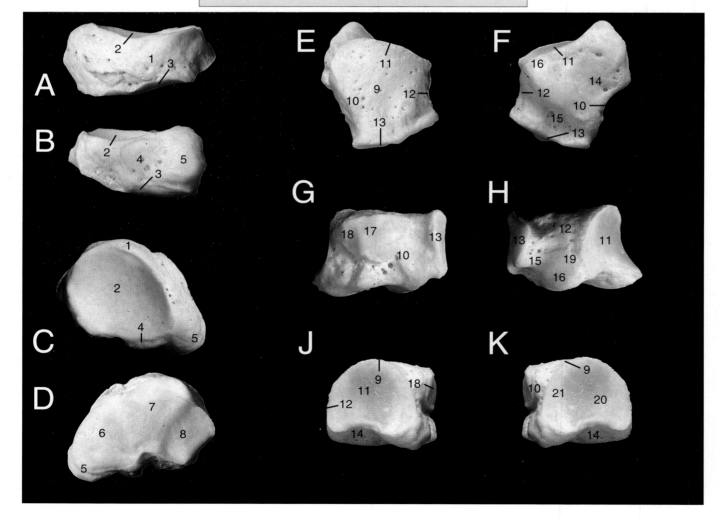

FOOT BONES
Articulated left cuneiform bones (medial, intermediate and lateral)
A From above
B From below
C Proximal (navicular) aspect (for distal aspect see page 63)

Left medial cuneiform bone
D From the medial side
E From the lateral side

1	Medial surface
2	Distal surface for first metatarsal
3	Area for tendon of tibialis anterior
4	Proximal surface for navicular
5	Lateral surface
6	Surface for second metatarsal
7	Surface for intermediate cuneiform
8	Area for peroneus longus tendon

Cuneiform bones
- Medial (the largest), intermediate (the smallest), and lateral.

- Situated between the navicular and the first three metatarsals.

Left intermediate cuneiform bone
F From the medial side
G From the lateral side

9	Medial surface
10	Surface for medial cuneiform
11	Distal surface for second metatarsal
12	Lateral surface
13	Surface for lateral cuneiform
14	Proximal surface for navicular

Left lateral cuneiform bone
H From the medial side
J From the lateral side

15	Medial surface
16	Surfaces for second metatarsal
17	Surface for intermediate cuneiform
18	Proximal surface for navicular
19	Lateral surface
20	Surface for cuboid
21	Surface for fourth metatarsal
22	Distal surface for third metatarsal

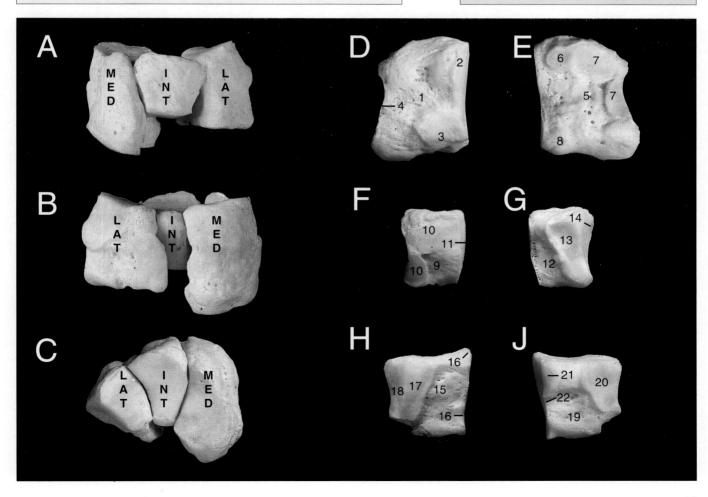

FOOT BONES
A and B Left metatarsal bones – numbered I-V with their medial and lateral sides named

The bones are arranged on their sides so that the articular surfaces on the adjacent sides of their bases can be seen

1 Groove on head for sesamoid bone	**10** Surface for fourth metatarsal
2 Surface for medial cuneiform	**11** Surface for third metatarsal
3 Area for bursa	**12** Surface for lateral cuneiform
4 Surface for medial cuneiform	**13** Surface for cuboid
5 Surface for intermediate cuneiform	**14** Surface for fifth metatarsal
6 Surfaces for third metatarsal	**15** Surface for fourth metatarsal
7 Surfaces for lateral cuneiform	**16** Surface for cuboid
8 Surfaces for second metatarsal	**17** Tuberosity of base
9 Surface for lateral cuneiform	

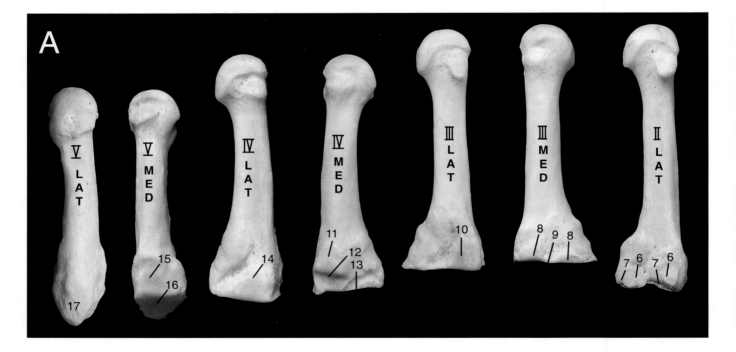

Metatarsal bones:

- First to fifth, leading to each toe and each with a base (at the proximal or ankle end), body or shaft, and head (at the toe end).
  Bases of first three articulate with cuneiform bones; bases of fourth and fifth articulate with the cuboid. Heads articulate with bases of proximal phalanges.

- The second, third and fourth metatarsals are longer than the first and fifth; the first is the shortest and the thickest.

- Refer to an articulated foot (page 40) and note the following:
  The base of the first metatarsal articulates with the medial cuneiform. There is normally a bursa but not a joint between the bases of the first and second metatarsals.
  The base of the second metatarsal articulates with all three cuneiforms and with the base of the third metatarsal. This second metatarsal base extends more proximally than the first and third bases – an interlocking device that prevents side-to-side movement.

FOOT BONES
C Left metatarsal bones – articulated, from above and behind

The metatarsal bones are articulated with each other but have been disarticulated from the cuneiform and cuboid bones, which have been rotated to show the surfaces that articulate with the metatarsals.

1 Surface of medial cuneiform for first metatarsal
2 Surface of intermediate cuneiform for second metatarsal
3 Surface of lateral cuneiform for third metatarsal
4 Surface of cuboid for fourth metatarsal
5 Surface of cuboid for fifth metatarsal

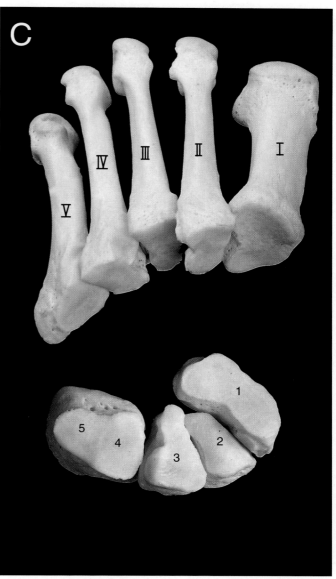

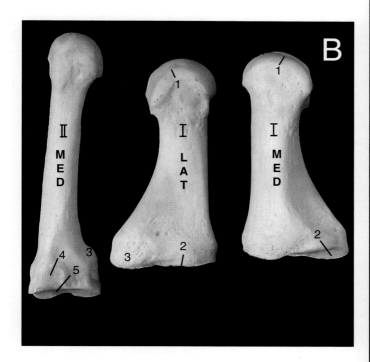

The base of the third metatarsal articulates with the lateral cuneiform and the bases of the second and fourth metatarsals.
The base of the fourth metatarsal articulates with the lateral cuneiform and the cuboid and the base of the fifth metatarsal.
The base of the fifth metatarsal articulates with the cuboid and the base of the fourth metatarsal.

LOWER LEG AND FOOT
A Superficial vessels and nerves of the left lower leg and foot, from the front

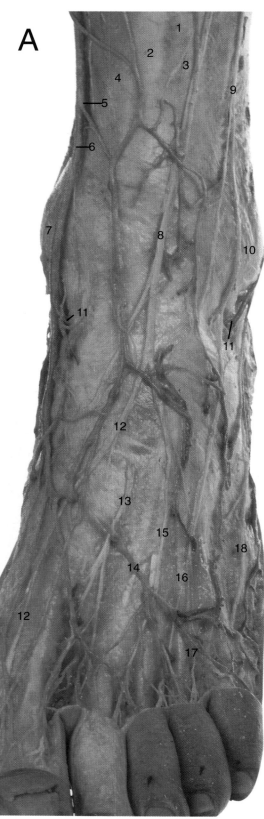

Skin and superficial connective tissue have been removed to show the superficial vessels and nerves lying on the deep fascia (1). In **A** the medial side of the dorsal venous arch (14) joins the medial marginal vein of the foot to form the great saphenous vein (5), which runs up in front of the medial malleolus (7). The medial and lateral branches of the superficial peroneal nerve (8 and 9) pass down on to the dorsum, supplemented on the medial side by the saphenous nerve (6) and on the lateral side by the sural nerve (18). The end of the deep peroneal nerve (13) perforates the deep fascia to run to the first toe cleft.

1	Deep fascia
2	Tendon of tibialis anterior (under fascia)
3	Tendon of extensor digitorum longus (under fascia)
4	Medial surface of tibia (under fascia)
5	Great saphenous vein
6	Saphenous nerve
7	Medial malleolus
8	Medial branch of superficial peroneal nerve
9	Lateral branch of superficial peroneal nerve
10	Lateral malleolus
11	A perforating vein
12	Proper dorsal digital nerve of great toe
13	Medial terminal branch of deep peroneal nerve
14	Dorsal venous arch
15	Dorsal digital nerve to second cleft
16	Dorsal digital nerve to third cleft
17	Dorsal digital nerve to fourth cleft
18	Sural nerve

- The skin of the first toe cleft is supplied by the *deep* peroneal nerve (**A13**); the skin of the other clefts is supplied by the *superficial* peroneal nerve (**A8** and **9**).

- The skin behind the ankle and at the back of the heel is supplied on the medial side by the saphenous nerve (**A6**, from the femoral nerve) and the medial calcanean branches (**B8**) of the tibial nerve, and on the lateral side by the sural nerve (**B2**, also from the tibial nerve).

- The saphenous nerve (**A6**) on the medial side of the foot supplies skin as far forward as the metatarso-phalangeal joint of the great toe.

- The sural nerve (**A18**) on the lateral side of the foot supplies skin as far forward as the side of the fifth toe.

- The skin of the medial side of the dorsum of the foot, including the region of the medial malleolus, is part of the fourth lumbar dermatome (**Fig. 8,** page 111.) The fifth lumbar dermatome includes the rest of the dorsum, and the first sacral dermatome includes the lateral side of the foot and the lateral malleolar region.

- The *great* saphenous vein (**A5**) passes upwards *in front of the medial* malleolus (**A7**).

- The *small* saphenous vein (**B3**) passes upwards *behind the lateral* malleolus (**B11**).

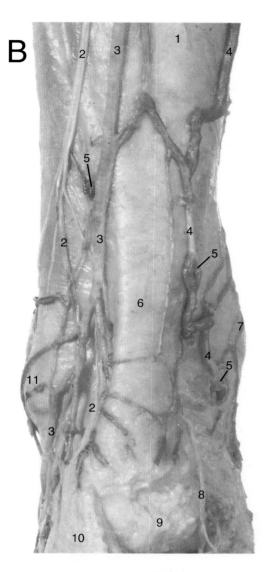

B

B Superficial vessels and nerves of the left lower leg and foot, from behind
C Cross section of the leg above the level of the upper part of B

In **B** the most obvious structure is the tendo calcaneus (Achilles' tendon, **6**), running down to be attached to the back of the calcaneus (**9**). The small saphenous vein (**3**) and sural nerve (**2**) with their tributaries and branches are behind the lateral malleolus (**11**). On both sides but especially the medial, there are some typical perforating veins (**5**), piercing the deep fascia to form communications between the superficial and deep veins. The posterior arch vein (**4**) unites several of the perforators on the medial side.

The section in **C** is viewed from below, looking from the ankle towards the knee. Tibialis posterior (**13**) is the deepest of the calf muscles (immediately behind the interosseous membrane, **5**), with the tibial nerve (**19**) behind it and the posterior tibial vessels (**20**) more medially, between flexor digitorum longus (**21**) and soleus (**14**). The peroneal artery (**12**) is adjacent to flexor hallucis longus (**11**) behind the fibula (**8**). Note the (unlabelled) dilated veins within and deep to soleus (**14**); they are the site for potentially dangerous deep venous thrombosis. In the anterior compartment, in front of the interosseous membrane (**5**), the anterior tibial vessels (**3**) and deep peroneal nerve (**4**) are between tibialis anterior (**2**) and extensor hallucis longus (**6**).

1 Deep fascia		fascia)
2 Sural nerve	**7**	Medial malleolus
3 Small saphenous vein	**8**	Medial calcanean nerve
4 Posterior arch vein	**9**	Posterior surface of calcaneus
5 A perforating vein	**10**	Fibrofatty tissue of heel
6 Tendo calcaneus (under	**11**	Lateral malleolus

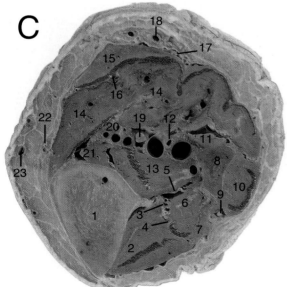

C

1	Tibia	**12**	Peroneal artery
2	Tibialis anterior	**13**	Tibialis posterior
3	Anterior tibial vessels	**14**	Soleus
4	Deep peroneal nerve	**15**	Gastrocnemius
5	Interosseous membrane	**16**	Plantaris tendon
6	Extensor hallucis longus	**17**	Sural nerve
7	Extensor digitorum longus	**18**	Small saphenous vein
8	Fibula	**19**	Tibial nerve
9	Superficial peroneal nerve	**20**	Posterior tibial vessels
10	Peroneus longus and brevis	**21**	Flexor digitorum longus
		22	Saphenous nerve
11	Flexor hallucis longus	**23**	Great saphenous vein

LOWER LEG AND FOOT

A Superficial vessels and nerves of the left lower leg and foot, from the medial side

This medial view emphasizes the position of the great saphenous vein (**3**) in front of the medial malleolus (**5**), with branches of the saphenous nerve (**4**) lying both in front of and behind the

vein. There are perforating veins (**9**) behind the malleolus and joining the posterior arch vein (**12**), and a large medial calcanean branch (**10**) of the tibial nerve running down to the skin of the heel.

1 Deep fascia
2 Medial surface of tibia
3 Great saphenous vein
4 Saphenous nerve
5 Medial malleolus
6 Dorsal venous arch
7 Proper dorsal digital nerve of great toe
8 Abductor hallucis (under fascia)
9 A perforating vein
10 Medial calcanean nerve
11 Tendo calcaneus (under fascia)
12 Posterior arch vein

- In the specimen shown on pages 64–67 some of the superficial veins are rather dilated and tortuous, but this has served to emphasize the posterior arch vein and perforating veins.

- The perforating veins (**A9**, **B8**) serve as communications between the superficial veins (above the deep fascia) and deep veins (below the fascia). Many of these communicating vessels possess valves that direct the flow of blood from superficial to deep; venous return from the limb is then brought about by the pumping action of the muscles (which are all below the deep fascia). If the valves become incompetent or the deep veins are blocked, pressure in the superficial veins increases and they become varicose (from the Latin for an enlarged and tortuous vessel).

- Perforating veins are variable in number and position but the most constant in the lower leg (**A9**) are near the posterior border of the tibia, one just below and one just above the medial malleolus (**A5**). The posterior arch vein (**A12**) unites these and perhaps other perforators and drains usually into the great saphenous vein below the knee.

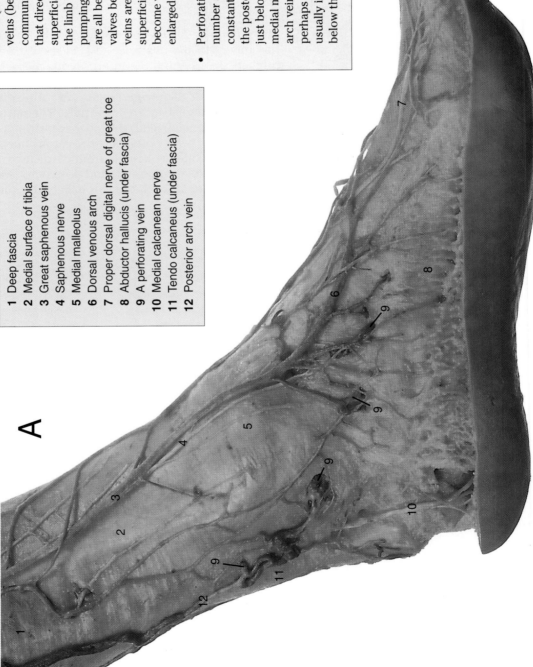

A

LOWER LEG AND FOOT
B Superficial vessels and nerves of the left lower leg and foot, from the lateral side

The medial and lateral branches of the superficial peroneal nerve (**1** and **2**) run on to the dorsum of the foot. Behind the lateral malleolus (**7**) are the small saphenous vein (**5**) and sural nerve (**4**). The tendon of peroneus longus (**3**) shines through the deep fascia above the malleolus.

1 Medial branch of superficial peroneal nerve
2 Lateral branch of superficial peroneal nerve
3 Deep fascia over peroneus longus tendon
4 Sural nerve
5 Small saphenous vein
6 Tendo calcaneus (under fascia)
7 Lateral malleolus
8 A perforating vein
9 Extensor digitorum brevis (under fascia)
10 Lateral marginal vein
11 Abductor digiti minimi (under fascia)
12 Dorsal venous arch

- The superficial veins of the dorsum include dorsal digital and dorsal metatarsal veins which join a dorsal venous arch (**B12**). The ends of the arch join medial and lateral marginal veins that run upwards to become the great and small saphenous veins respectively. (In **A** there is no obvious medial marginal vein, but there is a lateral marginal vein in **B,10**.)

- The deep veins run with the deep arteries. The larger arteries in the leg are usually accompanied by a pair of veins (venae commitantes).

- Lymph vessels, resembling narrow, thin-walled veins, accompany many arteries and veins, both superficial and deep. There are no lymph nodes in the foot; most of the lymphatic drainage of the lower limb is to inguinal nodes, but some lymphatic vessels drain into six or seven nodes that lie in the fat of the popliteal fossa. (Occasionally there is a single node beside the upper end of the anterior tibial artery in front of the interosseous membrane.)

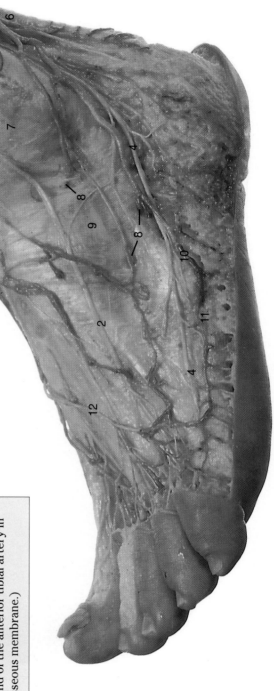

DEEP FASCIA OF THE FOOT
Deep fascia of the right lower leg and foot, from the front and the right

All superficial tissues, including vessels and nerves, have been removed to dispaly the deep fascia. It is thickened in places to form the retinacula (**2**, **4** - see notes) which keep tendons in their proper places; compare with the dissections on pages 70-73 where the fascia has been removed to leave only the retinacula. Here, with all the deep fascia intact, tendons and muscles can be seen shining through it.

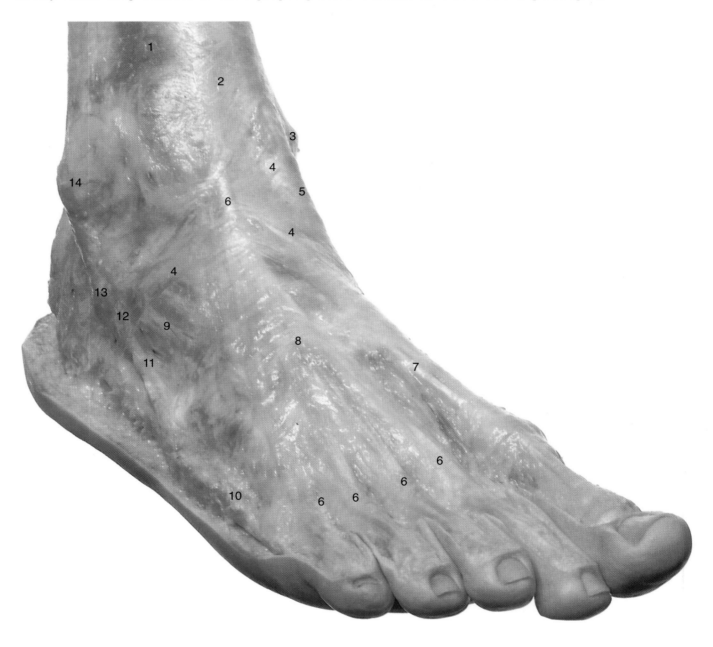

1 Deep fascia of leg	**8** Deep fascia of dorsum of foot
2 Superior extensor retinaculum	**9** Extensor digitorum brevis
3 Medial malleolus	**10** Abductor digiti minimi
4 Inferior extensor retinaculum	**11** Tendon of peroneus brevis
5 Tendon of tibialis anterior	**12** Inferior peroneal retinaculum
6 Tendons of extensor digitorum longus	**13** Tendon of peroneus longus
7 Tendon of extensor hallucis longus	**14** Lateral malleolus

- The retinacula of the ankle and foot are localized thickenings of deep fascia which keep tendons in place.

- There are two extensor retinacula (superior and inferior), a flexor retinaculum, and two peroneal retinacula (superior and inferior).

- The superior extensor retinaculum (**2**) is a band about 4cm broad, and is attached to the lower ends of the anterior borders of the tibia and fibula (see pages 70, **A7** and 72, **A12**).

- The inferior extensor retinaculum (**4**) is shaped like a letter Y lying on its side (see pages 70, **A9** and 72, **A13** and **B15**).
  The common stem of the Y is on the lateral side and is attached to the upper surface of the calcaneus in front of the sulcus calcanei. The tendons of extensor digitorum longus and peroneus tertius (with a common synovial sheath) pass beneath it.

The upper band of the Y continues upwards and medially from the common stem over the deep peroneal nerve and anterior tibial vessels, then forms a loop to enclose the extensor hallucis longus tendon (within a synovial sheath), finally becoming attached to the medial malleolus after passing either superficial or deep to the tendon of tibialis anterior (within a synovial sheath).
The lower band of the Y continues downwards and medially from the common stem, passing over the terminal branches of the deep peroneal nerve, the dorsalis pedis vessels and the tendons of extensor hallucis longus (within a syovial sheath) and tibialis anterior, to blend with the plantar aponeurosis overlying abductor hallucis.

- For the flexor retinaculum, see page 72.

- For the peroneal retinacula, see page 73.

DORSUM AND BACK OF THE FOOT
A Superficial dissection of the right lower leg and dorsum of the foot, from the front

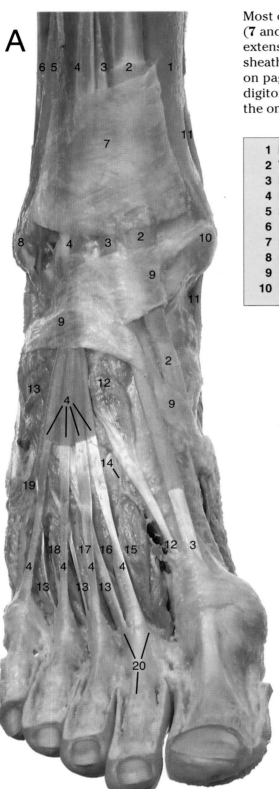

Most of the deep fascia has been removed, leaving only the retinacula (**7** and **9**). The most prominent structures are the long tendons of the extensor muscles (**2**, **3** and **4**) running down from the leg; the synovial sheaths surrounding the tendons in this specimen (which is also shown on pages 72 and 73) have been emphasized by blue tissue. Extensor digitorum brevis (**13**, with extensor hallucis brevis, **12** - see notes) is the only muscle to arise on the dorsum of the foot.

1	Medial surface of tibia	**11**	Tibialis posterior
2	Tibialis anterior	**12**	Extensor hallucis brevis
3	Extensor hallucis longus	**13**	Extensor digitorum brevis
4	Extensor digitorum longus	**14**	Dorsalis pedis artery
5	Subcutaneous surface of fibula	**15**	First dorsal interosseus
6	Peroneus brevis	**16**	Second dorsal interosseus
7	Superior extensor retinaculum	**17**	Third dorsal interosseus
8	Lateral malleolus	**18**	Fourth dorsal interosseus
9	Inferior extensor retinaculum	**19**	Peroneus tertius
10	Medial malleolus	**20**	Dorsal digital expansion

- Extensor digitorum longus (**4**) has four tendons which pass to the second, third, fourth and fifth toes.

- Extensor digitorum brevis (**13**) has four tendons which pass to the great, second, third and fourth toes. The part of the muscle that serves the great toe is known as extensor hallucis brevis (**12**).

- The dorsal digital expansions (extensor expansions, **20**) are derived from the tendons of extensor digitorum longus (**4**) as they pass over the metatarsophalangeal joints on to the dorsum of the proximal phalanges. They are each triangular in shape with the apex directed distally.
  On the second, third and fourth toes the basal angles of the expansions receive tendons from two interossei and one lumbrical muscle, and the central part of the base receives a tendon of extensor digitorum brevis (**13**). On the fifth toe one interosseus and one lumbrical tendon are attached.
  The central part of the apex is inserted into the base of the middle phalanx, while two collateral parts run farther forward to be inserted into the base of the distal phalanx (see page 42, **A16** and **17**).

- The order of the structures that pass beneath the superior extensor retinaculum and in front of the ankle joint from the medial to the lateral side is:
  Tibialis anterior tendon (with a synovial sheath) (**2**)
  Extensor hallucis longus tendon (with no synovial sheath) (**3**)
  Anterior tibial artery and venae comitantes ⎤ hidden between
  Deep peroneal nerve ⎦ **3** and **4**
  Extensor digitorum longus tendon (with no synovial sheath) (**4**)
  Peroneus tertius tendon (with no synovial sheath) (hidden by **4**)

DORSUM AND BACK OF THE FOOT
B Superficial dissection of the back of the right lower leg and foot

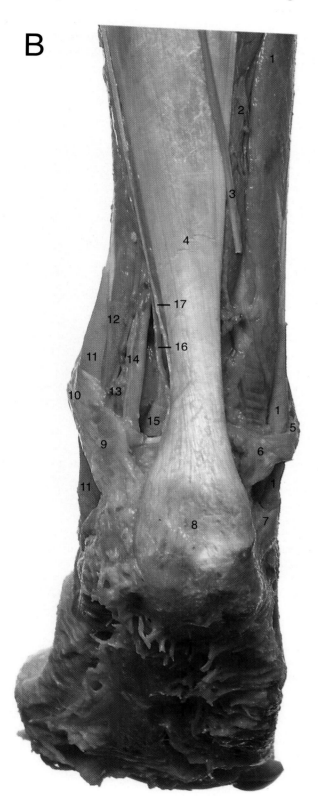

B

The deep fascia has been removed, leaving only the flexor and peroneal retinacula (**9, 6** and **7**). The Achilles' tendon (**4**) passes down to the back of the calcaneus (**8**). Flexor tendons (**11, 12** and **15**) lie behind the medial malleolus (**10**) and peroneal tendons (**1**) behind the lateral malleolus (**5**).

1	Peroneus longus overlapping peroneus brevis
2	Soleus
3	Sural nerve
4	Tendo calcaneus (Achilles' tendon)
5	Lateral malleolus
6	Superior peroneal retinaculum
7	Inferior peroneal retinaculum
8	Posterior surface of calcaneus
9	Flexor retinaculum
10	Medial malleolus
11	Tibialis posterior
12	Flexor digitorum longus
13	Posterior tibial artery and venae comitantes
14	Tibial nerve
15	Flexor hallucis longus
16	Medial calcanean nerve
17	Plantaris tendon

For the order of the structures behind the medial malleolus, see the notes on the flexor retinaculum on page 72.

DORSUM AND SIDES OF THE FOOT
A Superficial dissection of the right lower leg and foot, from the medial side.

The synovial sheaths of tendons have been emphasised by blue tissue. The deep fascia has been removed, leaving the flexor retinaculum (**12**), with part of the inferior extensor retinaculum (**15**) also visible in this view. The posterior tibial vessels (**4**) and the tibial nerve (**5**) lie between the tendons of flexor digitorum longus (**3**) in front and flexor hallucis longus (**6**) behind. The prominent muscle on the medial side of the sole is abductor hallucis (**14**).

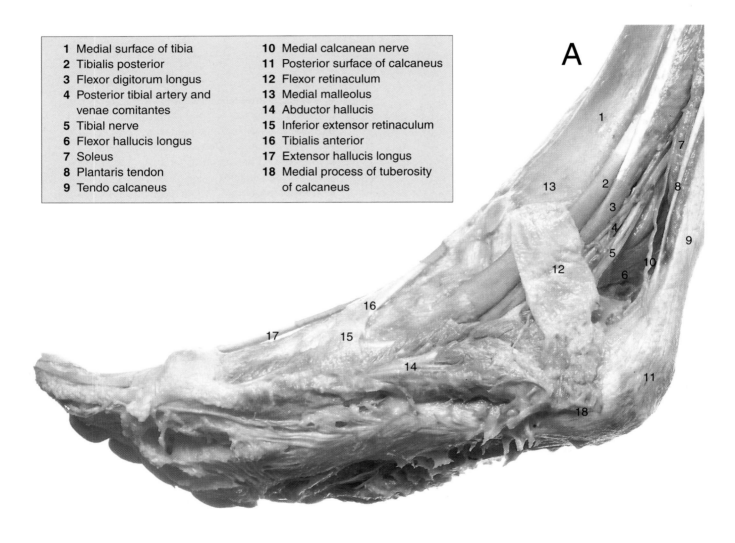

1	Medial surface of tibia	**10**	Medial calcanean nerve
2	Tibialis posterior	**11**	Posterior surface of calcaneus
3	Flexor digitorum longus	**12**	Flexor retinaculum
4	Posterior tibial artery and	**13**	Medial malleolus
	venae comitantes	**14**	Abductor hallucis
5	Tibial nerve	**15**	Inferior extensor retinaculum
6	Flexor hallucis longus	**16**	Tibialis anterior
7	Soleus	**17**	Extensor hallucis longus
8	Plantaris tendon	**18**	Medial process of tuberosity
9	Tendo calcaneus		of calcaneus

- The flexor retinaculum (**12**) passes from the medial malleolus to the medial process of the tuberosity of the calcaneus (**18**).
  Deep to the retinaculum are four connective tissue compartments – three for tendons and one for neurovascular structures. The order of the structures behind the medial malleolus from before backwards is:
  Tibialis posterior tendon (**2**, within a synovial sheath)
  Flexor digitorum longus tendon (**3**, within a synovial sheath)
  Posterior tibial artery and venae comitantes (**4**)
  Tibial nerve (**5**)
  Flexor hallucis longus tendon (**6**, within a synovial sheath).

DORSUM AND SIDES OF THE FOOT
B Superficial dissection of the right lower leg and foot, from the lateral side.

The synovial sheaths of tendons have been emphasized by blue tissue. The two extensor retinacula (**12** and **13**) and the two peroneal retinacula (**14** and **15**) have been preserved. The tendon of peroneus brevis (**4**) runs down to the fifth metatarsal, while that of peroneus longus (**5**) disappears to pass into the sole. Extensor digitorum brevis (**16**) forms a fleshy mass on the lateral side of the dorsum, and is crossed by the tendons of extensor digitorum longus (**3**) and peroneus tertius (**17**).

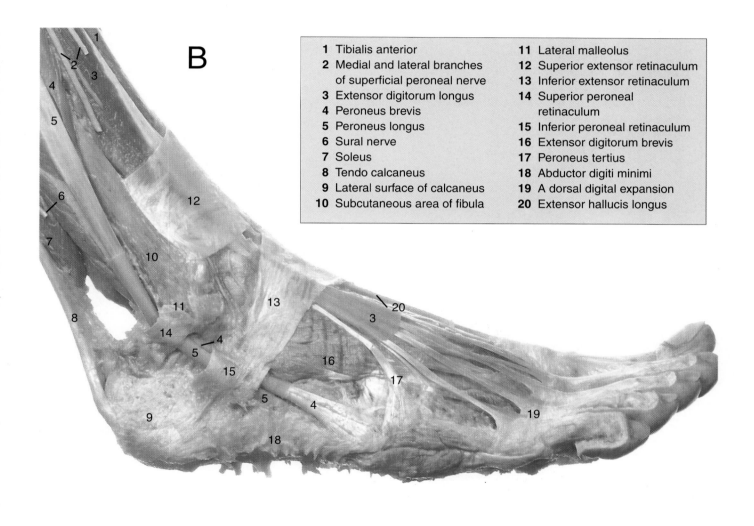

B

1 Tibialis anterior	**11** Lateral malleolus
2 Medial and lateral branches of superficial peroneal nerve	**12** Superior extensor retinaculum
3 Extensor digitorum longus	**13** Inferior extensor retinaculum
4 Peroneus brevis	**14** Superior peroneal retinaculum
5 Peroneus longus	**15** Inferior peroneal retinaculum
6 Sural nerve	**16** Extensor digitorum brevis
7 Soleus	**17** Peroneus tertius
8 Tendo calcaneus	**18** Abductor digiti minimi
9 Lateral surface of calcaneus	**19** A dorsal digital expansion
10 Subcutaneous area of fibula	**20** Extensor hallucis longus

- The superior peroneal retinaculum (**14**) passes from the lateral malleolus (**11**) to the lateral surface of the calcaneus (**9**).
  Deep to the retinaculum are the tendons of peroneus brevis (**4**) and peroneus longus (**5**) (both within a single synovial sheath). The brevis tendon is in front of the longus tendon.

- The inferior peroneal retinaculum (**15**) continues backwards and downwards from the common stem of the inferior extensor retinaculum (**13**) to the lateral surface of the calcaneus (**9**), with an intermediate attachment to the peroneal trochlea (see page 58, **D9**).
  Deep to the retinaculum above and in front of the trochlea is the peroneus brevis tendon (**4**, within its own synovial sheath), while below and behind the trochlea is the peroneus longus tendon (**5**, within its own synovial sheath).

DORSUM AND SIDES OF THE FOOT
Deep nerves and vessels of the right foot, from the front and right

The retinacula and most of the extensor tendons have been removed. The anterior tibial artery (11) of the leg continues into the dorsum as the dorsalis pedis artery (14), accompanied by the deep peroneal nerve (12 and 13). The lowest part of the anterior tibial artery gives off medial and lateral tarsal branches (24), and the dorsalis pedis gives off the arcuate artery (17) and the first dorsal metatarsal artery (15).

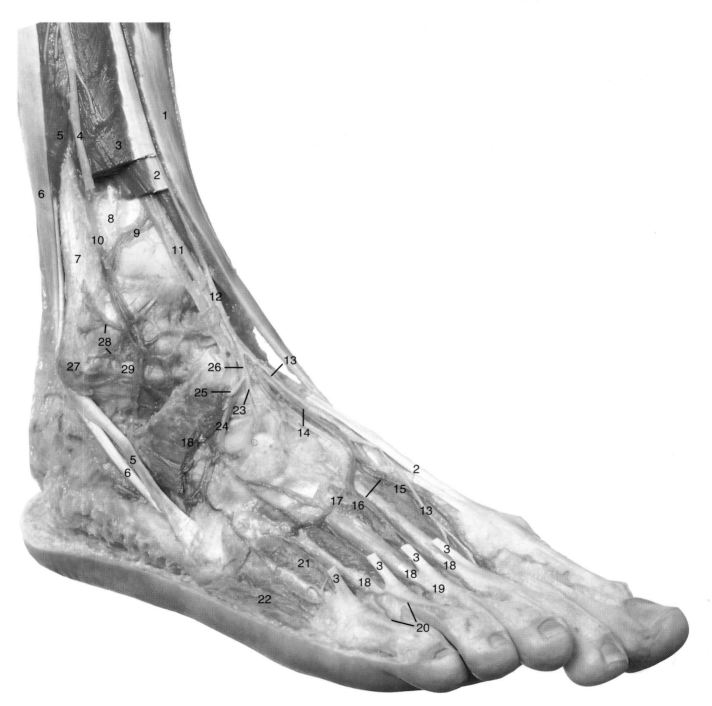

1 Tibialis anterior
2 Extensor hallucis longus
3 Extensor digitorum longus
4 Lateral branch of superficial peroneal nerve
5 Peroneus brevis
6 Peroneus longus
7 Subcutaneous surface of fibula
8 Interosseous membrane
9 Lateral malleolar artery and venae comitantes
10 Perforating branch of peroneal artery
11 Anterior tibial vessels
12 Deep peroneal nerve
13 Medial terminal branch of **12**
14 Dorsalis pedis artery
15 First dorsal metatarsal artery
16 Deep plantar artery
17 Arcuate artery
18 Extensor digitorum brevis (hallucis brevis to great toe)
19 Dorsal digital expansion
20 Dorsal digital artery
21 Fourth dorsal interosseus
22 Abductor digiti minimi
23 Interosseous branch of **26**
24 Lateral tarsal vessels
25 Nerve to extensor digitorum brevis
26 Lateral terminal branch of **12**
27 Lateral malleolus
28 Lateral malleolar arterial rete
29 Anterior talofibular ligament

- As the anterior tibial artery (**11**) crosses the lower margin of the tibia at the ankle joint it becomes the dorsalis pedis artery (**14**).

- After giving off medial and lateral tarsal branches (**24**) the dorsalis pedis artery (**14**) ends by dividing into the first dorsal metatarsal and the arcuate arteries (**15** and **17**).

- The first dorsal metatarsal artery (**15**) gives off a deep plantar (perforating) branch (**16**) that passes into the sole between the two heads of the first dorsal interosseus muscle to complete the plantar arch with the deep part of the lateral plantar artery (see page 81, **B18**).

- The arcuate artery (**17**) gives off the other three dorsal metatarsal arteries, and all the metatarsal arteries give dorsal digital branches.

- Sometimes the perforating branch of the peroneal artery (**10**), which anastomoses with the lateral tarsal and arcuate arteries (**24** and **17**), is large and replaces the dorsalis pedis artery, which is absent in about 12% of feet.

- Theoretically each side of each toe has a dorsal digital artery and a plantar digital artery but the individual vessels soon become merged into an anastomotic network.

- For a summary of the branches of the dorsalis pedis artery see page 113.

DEEP DISSECTION OF THE DORSUM
Joints beneath the talus of the left foot

The talus has been removed from the left foot and turned upside down to lie adjacent, so exposing the reciprocal joint surfaces. At the back the concave posterior articular surface of the talus (**27**) forms the talocalcanean joint with the convex posterior articular surface of the calcaneus (**9**). At the front are the various parts of the talocalcaneonavicular joint (see notes). The convex middle and anterior surfaces of the talus (**28** and **29**) articulate with the concave middle and anterior surfaces of the calcaneus (**13** and **14**), with part of the anterior surface of the talus (**30**) articulating with cartilage in the upper surface of the spring ligament (**15**). The convex head of the talus (**31**) articulates with the concave posterior surface of the navicular bone (**17**).

1 Tendo calcaneus
2 Bursa
3 Flexor hallucis longus
4 Lateral plantar nerve
5 Posterior tibial vessels
6 Medial plantar nerve
7 Flexor digitorum longus
8 Tibialis posterior
9 Posterior articular surface of calcaneus
10 Interosseous talocalcanean ligament
11 Inferior extensor retinaculum
12 Cervical ligament
13 Middle ⎤ articular surface
14 Anterior ⎦ of calcaneus
15 Cartilage in plantar calcaneonavicular (spring) ligament
16 Medial (deltoid) ligament of ankle joint
17 Posterior articular surface of navicular
18 Great saphenous vein
19 Tibialis anterior
20 Extensor hallucis longus
21 Deep peroneal nerve
22 Dorsalis pedis artery
23 Extensor digitorum longus
24 Extensor digitorum brevis
25 Peroneus brevis
26 Peroneus longus
27 Posterior ⎤ calcanean
28 Middle ⎬ articular surface
29 Anterior ⎦ of talus
30 Surface for plantar calcaneonavicular (spring) ligament
31 Surface for navicular

- Apart from the joints of the toes, the most important joints of the rest of the foot are those related to the talus.

- Above the talus is the ankle joint (properly known as the talocrural joint), between the trochlear surface of the talus and the lower ends of the tibia and fibula.

- Below the talus there are two separate joints. Towards the back is the talocalcanean joint (alternatively known as the subtalar joint – but see below), between the posterior articular surfaces of the lower part of the talus (**27**) and upper part of the calcaneus (**9**). In front is the talocalcaneonavicular joint, which is a two-part joint between the front of the head of the talus (**31**) and the navicular (**17**) (the talonavicular part of this joint), and the articulations of the under surface of the talus (**28–30**) with the anterior and middle facets on the upper surface of the calcaneus (**14** and **13**) and the upper surface of the plantar calcaneonavicular (spring) ligament (**15**) (the talocalcanean part of this joint).

- Unfortunately there is some confusion of terminology, for clinicians frequently use 'subtalar joint' as a collective name for *both* joints beneath the talus, not just the posterior one.

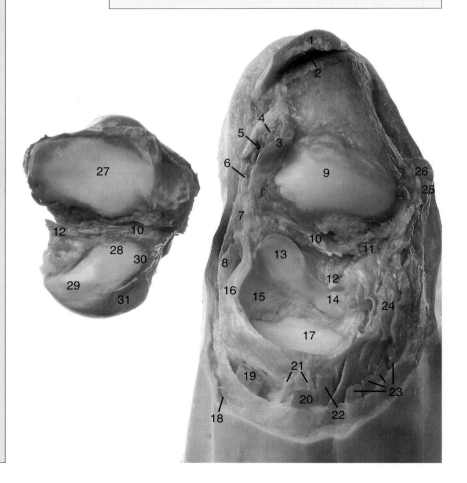

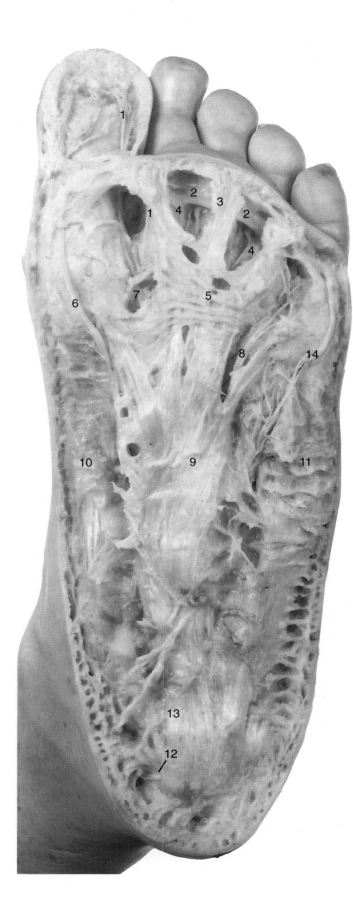

SOLE OF THE FOOT
Plantar aponeurosis of the left foot

Skin and subcutaneous tissue have been removed to show the thick central part of the plantar aponeurosis (**9**) and the thinner medial and lateral parts (**10** and **11**). The numerous strands and septa of fibrous tissue that attach the aponeurosis to the overlying tissues have not been removed to make a tidy dissection; they are an important part of the anatomy of the sole, binding adjacent tissues together.

1	Plantar digital nerve
2	Superficial transverse metatarsal ligament
3	Superficial layer of digital band of aponeurosis
4	Deep layer of digital band of aponeurosis
5	Transverse fibres of aponeurosis
6	Proper plantar digital nerve of great toe
7	Common plantar digital branch of medial plantar nerve
8	Common plantar digital branch of lateral plantar nerve
9	Central part of aponeurosis overlying flexor digitorum brevis
10	Medial part of aponeurosis overlying abductor hallucis
11	Lateral part of aponeurosis overlying abductor digiti minimi
12	Medial calcanean nerve
13	Medial process of tuberosity of calcaneus
14	Proper plantar digital nerve of fifth toe

- **Nerve supplies in the sole**
  Cutaneous: the medial plantar nerve supplies the medial part of the sole and the medial three and a half toes; the lateral plantar nerve supplies the lateral part of the sole and lateral one and a half toes.

  Muscular: the medial plantar nerve supplies abductor hallucis, flexor hallucis brevis, flexor digitorum brevis and the first lumbrical; the lateral plantar nerve supplies all the other small muscles of the sole.

  For details of nerve branches see pages 110 and 111.

- The skin under the heel and on the lateral part of the sole is part of the first sacral dermatome, with the fifth lumbar dermatome including the rest of the sole (**Fig. 8**, page 111).

- The superficial surface of the plantar aponeurosis is not smooth as in most textbook drawings, but roughened by the attachment of numerous fibrous septa forming loculations that hold the fatty subcutaneous tissues and skin in place when weight-bearing. They are well shown towards the back and sides of the dissection illustrated here.

SOLE OF THE FOOT
A First layer of muscles of the left sole

The plantar aponeurosis has been removed. The central muscle is flexor digitorum brevis (**19**), with abductor hallucis (**21**) on the medial side and abductor digiti minimi (**16**) on the lateral side. The most prominent tendon is that of flexor hallucis longus (**23**). Digital branches of the medial and lateral plantar nerves (**1, 2, 10, 11** and **14**) run forwards towards the toes, and the deep branch of the lateral plantar nerve (**17**) which supplies many of the deeper muscles curves deeply into the sole. See also **Fig. 3**, page 108.

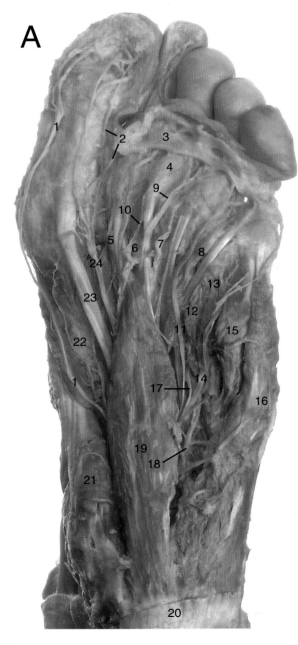

- The muscles of the sole are usually classified in *four layers*, as seen in progressively deep dissection:
  First layer : abductor hallucis (**A21**), flexor digitorum brevis (**A19**) and abductor digiti minimi (**A16**).
  Second layer : Flexor accessorius (**B19**) and the four lumbrical muscles (**B7-10**), with the tendons of flexor digitorum longus (**B4**) and flexor hallucis longus (**B1**).
  Third layer : flexor hallucis brevis (page 80, **A8**), adductor hallucis (page 80, **A6** and **7**) and flexor digiti minimi brevis (page 80, **A14**).
  Fourth layer : three plantar and four dorsal interosseus muscles (page 81, **B5-11**), with the tendons of tibialis posterior (page 81, **B27**) and peroneus longus (page 81, **B24**).
  The successive layers do not completely obscure one another; for example, the third plantar and fourth dorsal interossei (**A12** and **13**) are seen as soon as the plantar aponeurosis has been removed. (The layers refer to layers of *muscles*; the plantar aponeurosis is not itself the first layer but overlies it).

- It may be functionally more useful to classify the muscles into *medial, lateral and intermediate groups*:
  Medial group, for the great toe: abductor hallucis, flexor hallucis brevis, adductor hallucis and the tendon of flexor hallucis longus.
  Lateral group, for the fifth toe: abductor digiti minimi and flexor digiti minimi brevis.
  Intermediate group, for the second to fifth toes: flexor digitorum brevis, flexor accessorius, the tendons of flexor digitorum longus and the lumbricals, and the interossei.

1	Proper plantar digital nerve of great toe
2	Proper plantar digital nerves of first cleft
3	Superficial transverse metatarsal ligament
4	Fibrous flexor sheath
5	First lumbrical
6	Second lumbrical
7	Third lumbrical
8	Fourth lumbrical
9	Third plantar metatarsal artery
10	A superficial digital branch of medial plantar artery
11	Fourth common plantar digital nerve
12	Fourth dorsal interosseus
13	Third plantar interosseus
14	Proper plantar digital nerve of fifth toe
15	Flexor digiti minimi brevis
16	Abductor digiti minimi
17	Deep branch of lateral plantar nerve
18	Lateral plantar artery
19	Flexor digitorum brevis
20	Plantar aponeurosis
21	Abductor hallucis
22	Flexor hallucis brevis
23	Flexor hallucis longus
24	First common plantar digital nerve

SOLE OF THE FOOT
B Second layer of muscles of the left sole

Flexor digitorum brevis has been removed (but the abductors of the great and little toes, 27 and 16, remain) to display flexor accessorius (19) joining flexor digitorum longus (4) as it divides into its four tendons, from which the lumbrical muscles arise (7-10). The deep branch of the lateral plantar nerve (18) curls round the lateral side of flexor accessorius (19) to reach the deeper part of the sole, and numerous other muscular and digital (cutaneous) branches of the medial and lateral plantar nerves (26 and 22) are visible. Synovial sheaths of flexor tendons have been emphasized by blue tissue. See also **Fig. 4**, page 108.

- Although flexor hallucis longus (**B1**) passes to the great toe on the *medial* side of the foot, it arises from the *fibula* on the lateral side of the leg. The tendon crosses over in the sole, deep to flexor digitorum longus (**B4**, towards the back of the sole).

- The lateral and medial plantar nerves and vessels (**B20**, 22 and 26) pass between the first and second layers of muscles. The deep branch of the lateral plantar nerve (**A17**, **B18**) and the deep branch of the artery which becomes the lateral plantar arch (**B17**) curl deeply round the lateral border of flexor accessorius (**B19**).

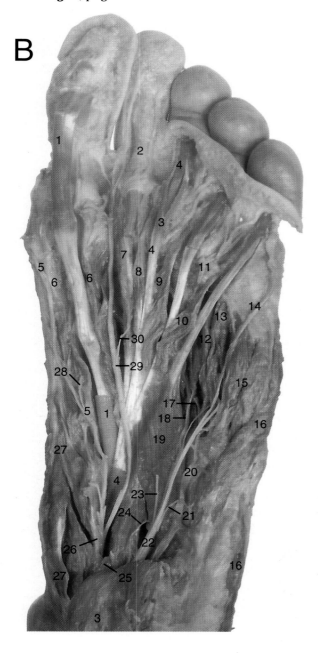

1	Flexor hallucis longus
2	Fibrous flexor sheath
3	Flexor digitorum brevis
4	Flexor digitorum longus
5	Proper plantar digital nerve of great toe
6	Flexor hallucis brevis
7	First lumbrical
8	Second lumbrical
9	Third lumbrical
10	Fourth lumbrical
11	Fourth plantar metatarsal artery
12	Fourth dorsal interosseus
13	Third plantar interosseus
14	Proper plantar digital nerve of fifth toe
15	Flexor digiti minimi brevis
16	Abductor digiti minimi
17	Plantar arch
18	Deep branch of lateral plantar nerve
19	Flexor accessorius
20	Lateral plantar artery
21	Nerve to abductor digiti minimi
22	Lateral plantar nerve
23	Fourth common plantar digital nerve
24	Nerve to flexor accessorius
25	Nerve to flexor digitorum brevis
26	Medial plantar artery overlying nerve
27	Abductor hallucis
28	Nerve to flexor hallucis brevis
29	First common plantar digital nerve
30	Nerve to first lumbrical

SOLE OF THE FOOT
A Third layer of muscles of the left sole

Most of the flexors and abductors have been re-moved, displaying the two heads of adductor hallucis (**6** and **7**), flexor hallucis brevis (**8**, which divides to pass to either side of the great toe), flexor digiti minimi brevis (**14**) and interossei (**9-11**). The deep branch of the lateral plantar nerve (**17**) is accompanied by the plantar arch (**16**) (from the lateral plantar artery, **19**). See also **Fig. 5**, page 109.

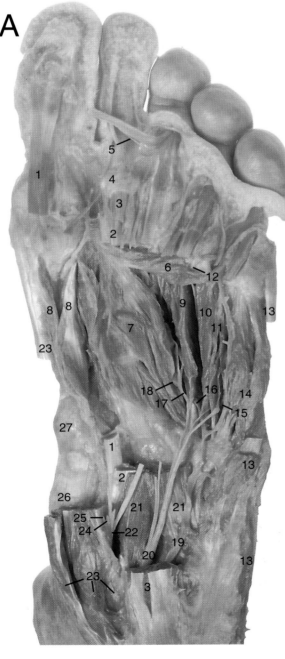

- For a summary of the medial and lateral plantar nerves see pages 110 and 111.

- The third common plantar digital nerve (from the medial plantar nerve) frequently has a communicating branch with the (fourth) common plantar digital branch of the lateral plantar nerve, but it was not present in the specimens dissected here.

- Branches of the lateral plantar nerve (**A20, B21**) to various interosseus muscles (**A9–11, B5–11**) can be seen but have been left unlabelled.

- The plantar arch (**B18**) is the deep continuation of the lateral plantar artery (**B20**), which is the larger terminal branch of the posterior tibial artery. The arch is completed by anastomosis with the deep plantar (perforating) branch of the first dorsal metatarsal artery (see page 74, **15**). The arch gives off four plantar metatarsal arteries (as in **B15** and **16**) which divide to give plantar digital branches to the sides of adjacent toes. There are separate branches for the medial side of the great toe and lateral side of the fifth toe.

- The medial plantar artery (**A24, B23**), smaller than the lateral and subject to considerable variation, does not take part directly in the formation of the arch. It ususally anastomoses with the plantar digital branch to the medial side of the great toe, and gives off superficial digital branches that anastomose with the first three plantar metatarsal arteries.

1 Flexor hallucis longus
2 Flexor digitorum longus
3 Flexor digitorum brevis
4 Fibrous flexor sheath
5 Long vinculum
6 Transverse head ⎤ of adductor hallucis
7 Oblique head ⎦
8 Flexor hallucis brevis
9 Second plantar interosseus
10 Fourth dorsal interosseus
11 Third plantar interosseus
12 Fourth plantar metatarsal artery
13 Abductor digiti minimi
14 Flexor digiti minimi brevis
15 Nerve to flexor digiti minimi brevis
16 Plantar arch
17 Deep branch of lateral plantar nerve
18 Nerve to adductor hallucis
19 Lateral plantar artery
20 Lateral plantar nerve
21 Flexor accessorius
22 Medial plantar nerve
23 Abductor hallucis
24 Medial plantar artery
25 Nerve to abductor hallucis
26 Tuberosity of navicular
27 Tibialis anterior

SOLE OF THE FOOT
B Fourth layer of muscles of the left sole

Most of the smaller muscles have been removed, leaving only the three plantar interossei (**7**, **9** and **11**) and the four dorsal interossei (**5**, **6**, **8** and **10**). The tendon of tibialis posterior (**27**) passes mainly to the tuberosity of the navicular (**26**), and the tendon of peroneus longus (**24**) crosses the sole obliquely from the lateral to the medial side. The end of the synovial sheath of flexor hallucis longus (**1**) has been emphasized by blue tissue. See also **Fig. 6**, page 109.

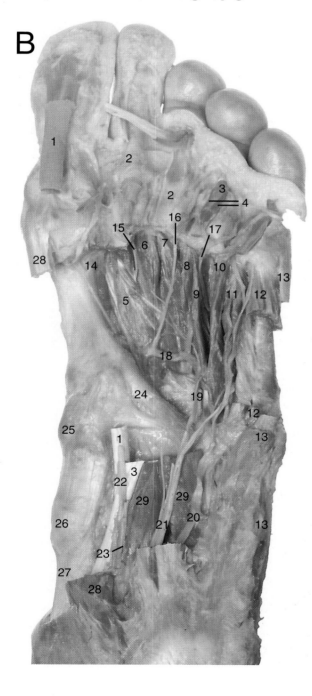

- Viewed from the sole, both plantar *and* dorsal interossei (**B5–11**) are visible; they lie side by side, not (as might be expected from their names) with the plantar group completely overlying and obscuring the dorsal. (But on the dorsum only dorsal interossei are seen between the metatarsals – as on page 70, **A15–18**.)
  The *p*lantar interossei *ad*duct toes and the *d*orsal interossei *ab*duct them at the metatarsophalangeal joints, the reference line or axis for these movements being the line of the second toe. The mnemonics PAD and DAB are the usual aids to recalling which group does what.
  The great toe and the fifth toe each have their own abductor muscle; the great toe also has its own adductor to draw it nearer the second toe. It follows that there must be a plantar interosseus for each of the third, fourth and fifth toes so that they can be adducted towards the axial line. The second toe has no plantar interosseus but it has two dorsal interossei, one on each side so that it can be abducted to either side of its own neutral position. The third and fourth toes both have one of each interosseus.

- For other and probably more important actions of the interossei see page 93.

- For a summary of the medial and lateral plantar arteries see page 114.

1	Flexor hallucis longus
2	Fibrous flexor sheath
3	Flexor digitorum longus
4	Flexor digitorum brevis
5	First dorsal ⎤
6	Second dorsal
7	First plantar
8	Third dorsal ├ interosseus
9	Second plantar
10	Fourth dorsal
11	Third plantar ⎦
12	Flexor digiti minimi brevis
13	Abductor digiti minimi
14	First plantar metatarsal artery
15	Second plantar metatarsal artery
16	Third plantar metatarsal artery
17	Fourth plantar metatarsal artery
18	Plantar arch
19	Deep branch of lateral plantar nerve
20	Lateral plantar artery
21	Lateral plantar nerve
22	Medial plantar nerve
23	Medial plantar artery
24	Peroneus longus
25	Tibialis anterior
26	Tuberosity of navicular
27	Tibialis posterior
28	Abductor hallucis
29	Flexor accessorius

LIGAMENTS OF THE FOOT
Ligaments of the right foot
A From the right and above
B From the lateral side
C From behind

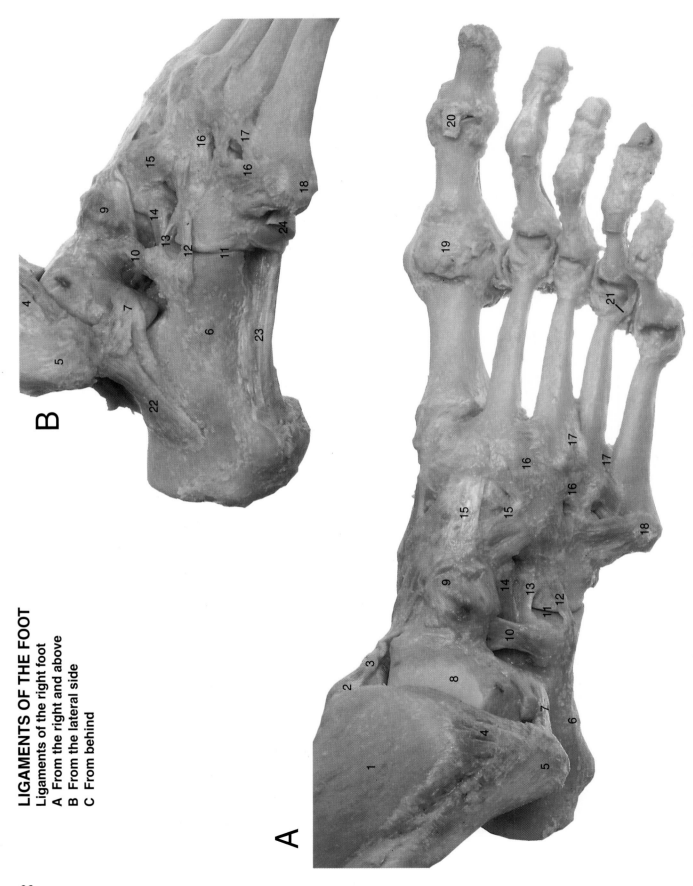

C

On the medial side of the ankle joint there is a single medial (deltoid) ligament (A3) (although it has several parts, as on page 84, A2–5), but on the lateral side there is no single lateral ligament but three separate ligaments: the anterior and posterior talofibular ligaments (A7 and B7, C28) and the calcaneofibular ligament (B22 and C22).

1 Tibia
2 Medial malleolus
3 Medial (deltoid) ligament of ankle joint
4 Anterior tibiofibular ligament
5 Lateral malleolus
6 Calcaneus
7 Anterior talofibular ligament
8 Trochlear surface of talus
   (ankle joint capsule removed)
9 Head of talus
   (under capsule of talonavicular part of talocalcaneonavicular joint)
10 Cervical ligament
11 Calcaneocuboid joint
12 Dorsal calcaneocuboid ligament
13 Calcaneocuboid part ⎤ of bifurcate
14 Calcaneonavicular part ⎦ ligament
15 Dorsal cuneonavicular ligaments
16 Dorsal tarsometatarsal ligaments
17 Dorsal metatarsal ligaments
18 Tuberosity of base of fifth metatarsal
19 Capsule of first metatarsophalangeal joint
20 Tendon of extensor hallucis longus
21 Collateral ligament
22 Calcaneofibular ligament
23 Long plantar ligament
24 Tendon of peroneus longus
25 Interosseous membrane
26 Posterior tibiofibular ligament
27 Tibial slip of 28
28 Posterior talofibular ligament
29 Groove for flexor hallucis longus tendon on talus and sustentaculum tali
30 Posterior tibiotalal part ⎤ of medial
31 Tibiocalcanean part ⎦ (deltoid) ligament
32 Groove for tibialis posterior tendon
33 Groove for peroneus brevis tendon

In **A** the foot is plantarflexed, showing part of the trochlear (superior articular) surface of the talus (**8**), with the front of the deltoid ligament (**3**) on the medial side and the anterior tibiofibular ligament (**4**) on the lateral side. The cervical ligament (**10**) passes upwards and medially from the upper surface of the calcaneus to the under surface of the talus, and in front of it are the two parts of the bifurcate ligament (**13** and **14**) with a small dorsal calcaneocuboid ligament (**12**) more laterally. Other dorsal ligaments (**15**, **16** and **17**) connect adjacent bones.

In **B** the anterior talofibular ligament (**7**) and calcaneofibular ligament (**22**) are seen, with some of the smaller dorsal ligaments (**12-17**), and so is the posterior part of the long plantar ligament (**23**) in the sole.

In **C** the posterior talofibular ligament (**28**) runs transversely (so it is not seen in the lateral view in **B**); it has a tibial slip (**27**) which merges with the inferior transverse ligament, the name given to the lower part of the posterior tibiofibular ligament (**26**).

LIGAMENTS OF THE FOOT

A Ligaments of the right foot, from the medial side

On the medial side of the ankle the various parts of the medial (deltoid) ligament (2-5) merge with one another. The tendon of tibialis posterior (7) is mainly attached to the tuberosity of the navicular (8), while that of tibialis anterior (13) runs to the medial cuneiform and the base of the first metatarsal.

1 Medial malleolus
2 Posterior tibiotalal part ⎤
3 Tibiocalcanean part   ⎥ of medial (deltoid) ligament
4 Anterior tibiotalal part ⎥
5 Tibionavicular part   ⎦
6 Sustentaculum tali
7 Tibialis posterior
8 Tuberosity of navicular
9 Long plantar ligament
10 Dorsal cuneonavicular ligament
11 Talonavicular ligament
12 Dorsal ligaments of first tarsometatarsal joint
13 Tibialis anterior
14 Capsule   ⎤
15 Collateral ligament ⎦ of first metatarsophalangeal joint
16 Sesamoid bone
17 Flexor hallucis longus
18 Collateral ligament of interphalangeal joint
19 Extensor hallucis longus

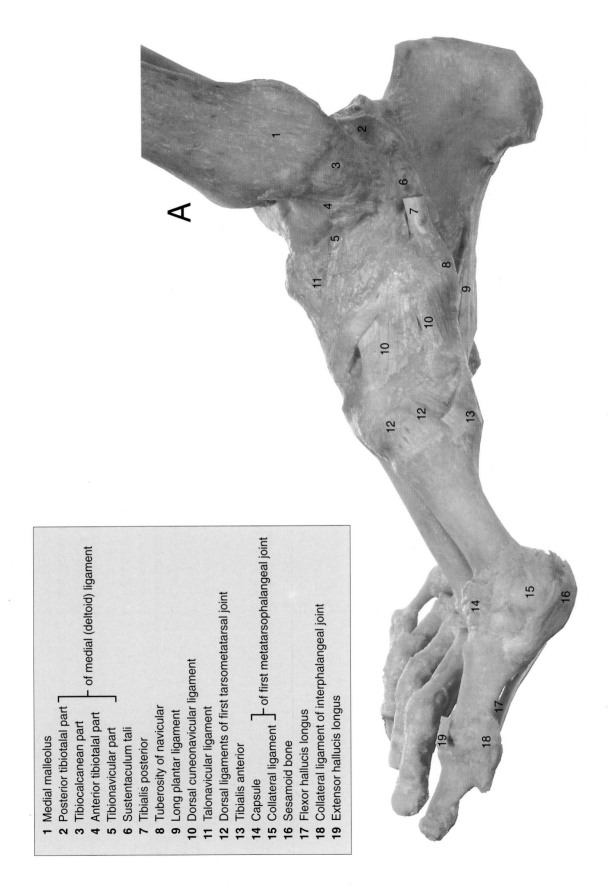

A

LIGAMENTS OF THE FOOT
B Ligaments of the sole of the right foot

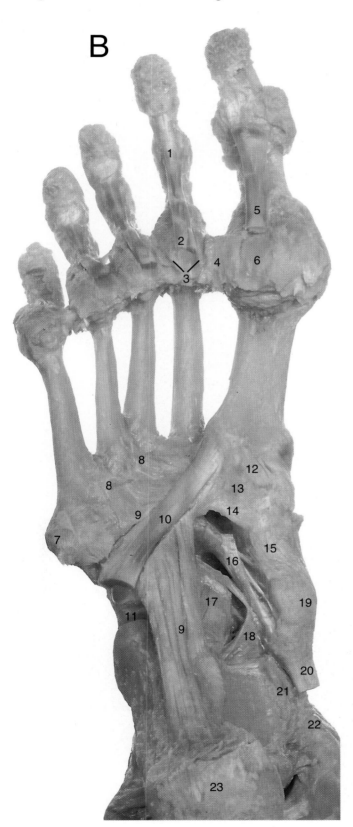

Part of the long plantar ligament (**9**) has been cut away to show the tendon of peroneus longus (**10**) lying in the groove on the cuboid. Medial to the posterior part of the long plantar ligament is the short plantar (plantar calcaneocuboid) ligament (**17**), and medial to that is the spring (plantar calcaneonavicular) ligament (**18**). At the anterior part of the foot the deep transverse metatarsal ligaments (**4**) keep the heads of the metatarsals and the bases of the toes from spreading apart.

 1 Flexor digitorum longus
 2 Flexor digitorum brevis
 3 Fibrous flexor sheath
 4 Deep transverse metatarsal ligament
 5 Flexor hallucis longus
 6 Plantar ligament of first tarsometatarsal joint
 7 Tuberosity of base of fifth metatarsal
 8 Plantar metatarsal ligaments
 9 Long plantar ligament
10 Tendon of peroneus longus in groove on cuboid
11 Calcaneocuboid joint
12 Plantar tarsometatarsal ligament
13 Medial cuneiform
14 Cuneometatarsal ligament
15 Plantar cuneonavicular ligament
16 Fibrous slip from tibialis posterior overlying a cuneometatarsal ligament
17 Plantar calcaneocuboid (short plantar) ligament
18 Plantar calcaneonavicular (spring) ligament
19 Tuberosity of navicular
20 Tendon of tibialis posterior
21 Sustentaculum tali and groove for flexor hallucis longus
22 Medial (deltoid) ligament of ankle joint
23 Tuberosity of calcaneus

- The *medial* sides of the medial cuneiform and the base of the first metatarsal receive the attachment of the tibialis anterior tendon (**A13**); the *lateral* sides of the same two bones receive the attachment of the peroneus longus tendon (**B10**).

- The plantar calcaneocuboid ligament (**B17**), commonly called the short plantar ligament, is largely under cover of the long plantar ligament (**B9**), which with the groove on the cuboid bone forms an osseofibrous tunnel for the peroneus longus tendon (**B10**).

- The plantar calcaneonavicular ligament (**B18**), passing from the sustentaculum tali of the calcaneus to the navicular and commonly called the spring ligament although it is not elastic, is an important support for the head of the talus in the talocalcaneonavicular joint (page 76, **15**).

SECTIONS AND IMAGES OF THE FOOT

Sagittal sections of the right foot

A Through the medial part of the talus, sustentaculum tali of the calcaneus and the great toe, from the lateral side

B Through the centre of the talus, medial part of the calcaneus and the great toe, from the lateral side (in a different foot from that in **A**)

1　Tibia
2　Tibialis posterior
3　Flexor digitorum longus
4　Tibial nerve
5　Flexor hallucis longus
6　Talus
7　Sustentaculum tali
8　Plantar calcaneonavicular (spring) ligament
9　Navicular
10　Tibialis anterior
11　Medial cuneiform
12　First metatarsal
13　Extensor hallucis longus
14　Proximal phalanx
15　Distal phalanx
16　Sesamoid bone
17　Flexor hallucis brevis
18　Proper plantar digital nerve of great toe
19　Abductor hallucis
20　Medial plantar nerve and vessels

In **A** the section passes through the metatarsal and phalanges of the great toe (**12, 14** and **15**) and the sustentaculum tali of the calcaneus (**7**); the section is too far medial to show any other part of the calcaneus. The plantar calcaneonavicular (spring) ligament (**8**) stretches between the sustentaculum (**7**) and the navicular, with the tendons of tibialis posterior (**2**) and flexor digitorum longus (**3**) giving support below the ligament. The bulky muscle below the sustentaculum is abductor hallucis (**19**). Note one of the sesamoid bones (**16**) beneath the head of the first metatarsal (**12**).

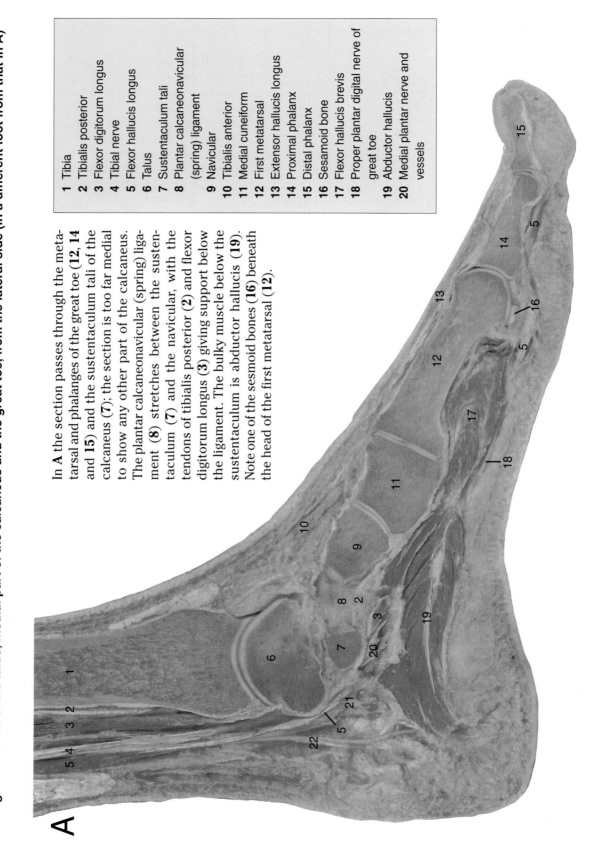

In **B** the section again passes through the bones of the great toe but more laterally, showing the two joints beneath the talus–the talocalcaneo-navicular joint (**27**) and the talocalcanean joint (**24**) – with the interosseous talocalcanean ligament (**25**) in between. The lowest part of the calcaneus is the medial process of the tuberosity (**38**). Note the bursa (**39**) between the Achilles' tendon and the upper part of the calcaneus, and the additional sesamoid bone (**33**) under the head of the first phalanx of the great toe.

For further details of the great toe see page 98.

21 Lateral plantar nerve and vessels
22 Medial calcanean nerve
23 Ankle joint
24 Talocalcanean joint
25 Interosseous talocalcanean ligament
26 Calcaneus
27 Talocalcanean part of talocalcaneonavicular joint
28 Talonavicular part of talocalcaneonavicular joint
29 Cuneonavicular joint
30 Cuneometatarsal joint
31 Metatarsophalangeal joint
32 Interphalangeal joint
33 Additional sesamoid bone
34 Peroneus longus
35 Plantar aponeurosis
36 Flexor accessorius
37 Abductor digiti minimi
38 Medial process of tuberosity of calcaneus
39 Bursa
40 Tendo calcaneus

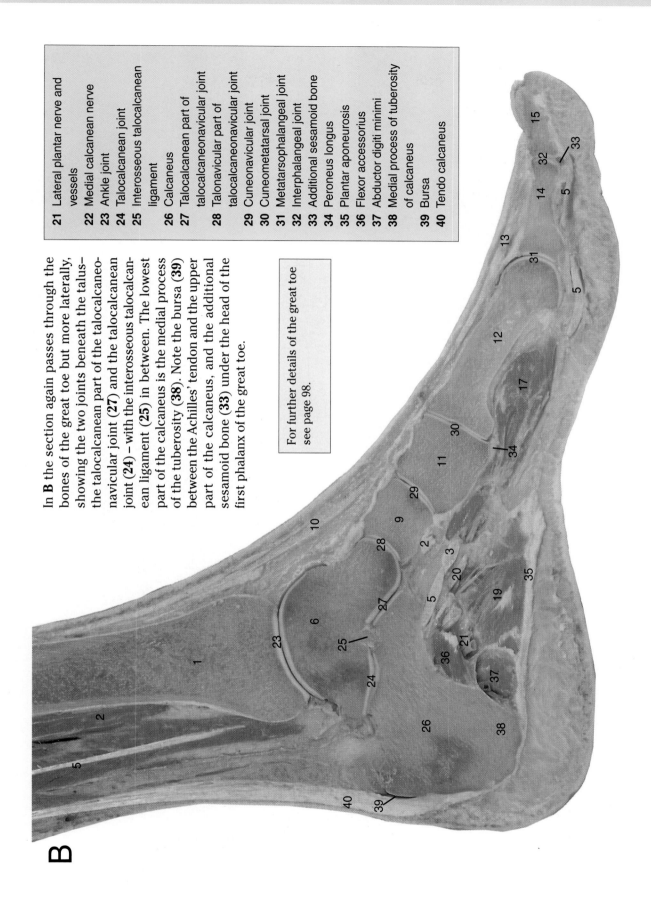

B

SECTIONS AND IMAGES OF THE FOOT

Sagittal sections of the right foot
A Through the second toe, from the lateral side
B Through the fifth toe, from the medial side

In **A** in the sagittal plane through the second metatarsal (**22**), small parts of the cuboid and medial cuneiform (**17** and **19**) lie underneath parts of the navicular and intermediate cuneiform (**16** and **18**). This is because of the shapes of the bones that form the transverse arch of the foot; compare with the view from below of the bones of the articulated foot on page 40, **B**. The thick plantar aponeurosis (**34**) overlies flexor digitorum brevis (**33**) with, towards the back, part of abductor digiti minimi (**37**), whose origin extends unexpectedly far medially.

1 Tibialis anterior
2 Extensor hallucis longus
3 Tibia
4 Tibialis posterior
5 Flexor hallucis longus
6 Tendo calcaneus
7 Ankle joint
8 Talus
9 Lateral tubercle of talus
10 Talocalcanean joint
11 Calcaneus
12 Interosseous talocalcanean ligament
13 Talocalcanean part of talocalcaneonavicular joint
14 Plantar calcaneonavicular (spring) ligament
15 Talonavicular part of talocalcaneonavicular joint
16 Navicular
17 Cuboid
18 Intermediate cuneiform
19 Medial cuneiform
20 Extensor digitorum brevis

A

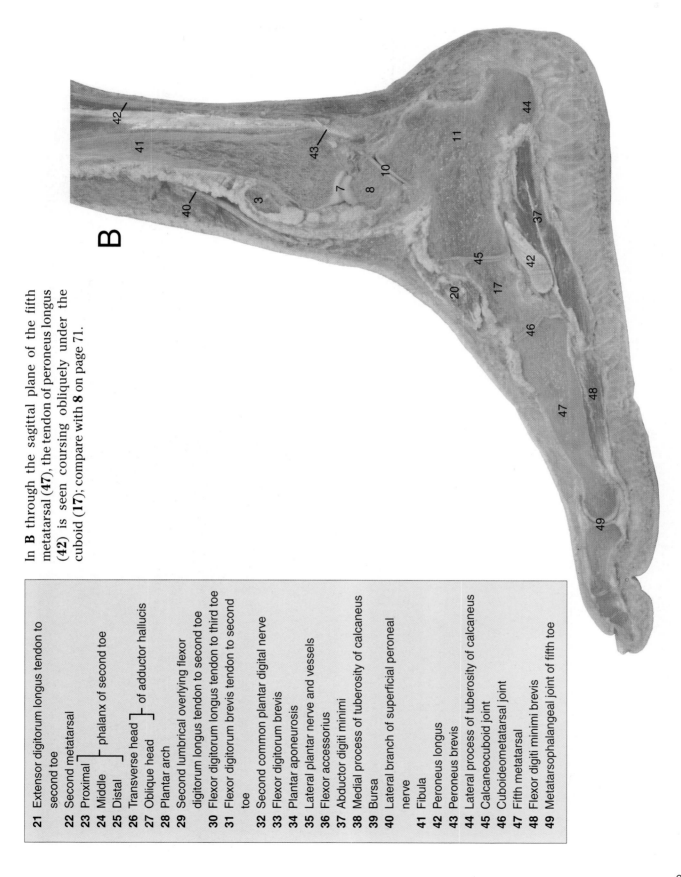

B

In **B** through the sagittal plane of the fifth metatarsal (**47**), the tendon of peroneus longus (**42**) is seen coursing obliquely under the cuboid (**17**); compare with **8** on page 71.

21 Extensor digitorum longus tendon to second toe
22 Second metatarsal
23 Proximal ⎱ phalanx of second toe
24 Middle ⎰ of second toe
25 Distal
26 Transverse head ⎱ of adductor hallucis
27 Oblique head ⎰
28 Plantar arch
29 Second lumbrical overlying flexor digitorum longus tendon to second toe
30 Flexor digitorum longus tendon to third toe
31 Flexor digitorum brevis tendon to second toe
32 Second common plantar digital nerve
33 Flexor digitorum brevis
34 Plantar aponeurosis
35 Lateral plantar nerve and vessels
36 Flexor accessorius
37 Abductor digiti minimi
38 Medial process of tuberosity of calcaneus
39 Bursa
40 Lateral branch of superficial peroneal nerve
41 Fibula
42 Peroneus longus
43 Peroneus brevis
44 Lateral process of tuberosity of calcaneus
45 Calcaneocuboid joint
46 Cuboideometatarsal joint
47 Fifth metatarsal
48 Flexor digiti minimi brevis
49 Metatarsophalangeal joint of fifth toe

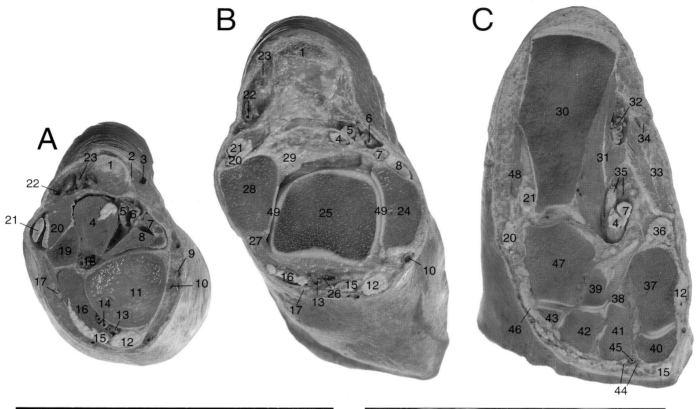

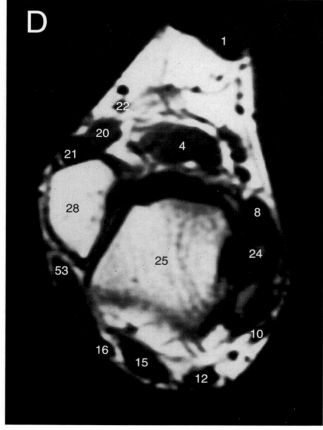

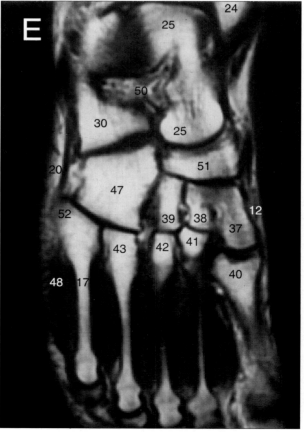

By courtesy of Dr Peter Abrahams

SECTIONS AND IMAGES OF THE FOOT
Sections and images of the right lower leg and foot
A Transverse section 6 cm above the ankle joint
B Transverse section through the ankle joint
C Oblique section 5 cm below the ankle joint
D Axial magnetic resonance (MR) image of the ankle joint
E Axial magnetic resonance (MR) image of the foot

Above the ankle in **A** peroneus brevis (**20**) is behind the fibula (**19**) with the tendon of peroneus longus (**21**) lying laterally, but at the lower levels in **B** and **C** the tendon of peroneus longus (**21**) is behind that of peroneus brevis (**20**). The lowest part of flexor hallucis longus (**4**) is seen arising from the fibula (**19**).

At the level of the medial malleolus (**24**) in **B**, the tendon of tibialis posterior (**8**) lies adjacent to the bone, with the tendon of flexor digitorum longus (**7**) immediately behind it. The posterior tibial vessels (**6**) and the tibial nerve (**5**) intervene between the digitorum tendon (**7**) and the tendon of flexor hallucis longus (**4**). At the front of the medial malleolus (**24**) in **B**, note the great saphenous vein (**10**), and in front of the talus (**25**) the dorsalis pedis artery (**26**) and deep peroneal nerve (**13**)

lie between the tendons of extensor hallucis longus (**15**) and extensor digitorum longus (**16**).

In the oblique section in **C** the cuboid (**47**) lies in front of the calcaneus (**30**), and at a lower level the tendon of peroneus longus (**21**) will pass underneath the cuboid. On the medial side behind the medial cuneiform (**37**) the very tip of the tuberosity of the navicular (**36**) receives the main attachment of tibialis posterior. The tendons of flexor hallucis longus (**4**) and flexor digitorum longus (**7**) are more laterally placed.

Compare the MR image in **D** with the section in **B**, and **E** with **C**; the images are at similar but not identical levels.

1 Tendo calcaneus	**28**	Lateral malleolus
2 Plantaris	**29**	Posterior talofibular ligament
3 A tributary of great saphenous vein	**30**	Calcaneus
4 Flexor hallucis longus	**31**	Flexor accessorius
5 Tibial nerve	**32**	Lateral plantar nerve and vessels
6 Posterior tibial vessels	**33**	Abductor hallucis
7 Flexor digitorum longus	**34**	Medial calcanean nerve
8 Tibialis posterior	**35**	Medial plantar nerve and vessels
9 Saphenous nerve	**36**	Tip of tuberosity of navicular and tibialis posterior
10 Great saphenous vein	**37**	Medial ⎤
11 Tibia	**38**	Intermediate ⊢ cuneiform
12 Tibialis anterior	**39**	Lateral ⎦
13 Deep peroneal nerve	**40**	First ⎤
14 Anterior tibial vessels	**41**	Second ⊢ metatarsal base
15 Extensor hallucis longus	**42**	Third
16 Extensor digitorum longus	**43**	Fourth ⎦
17 Superficial peroneal nerve	**44**	First dorsal interosseus
18 Peroneal vessels	**45**	Deep plantar artery
19 Fibula	**46**	Extensor digitorum brevis
20 Peroneus brevis	**47**	Cuboid
21 Peroneus longus	**48**	Abductor digiti minimi
22 Small saphenous vein	**49**	Ankle joint
23 Sural nerve	**50**	Tarsal sinus
24 Medial malleolus	**51**	Navicular
25 Talus	**52**	Tuberosity of base of fifth metatarsal
26 Dorsalis pedis artery	**53**	Peroneus tertius
27 Anterior talofibular ligament		

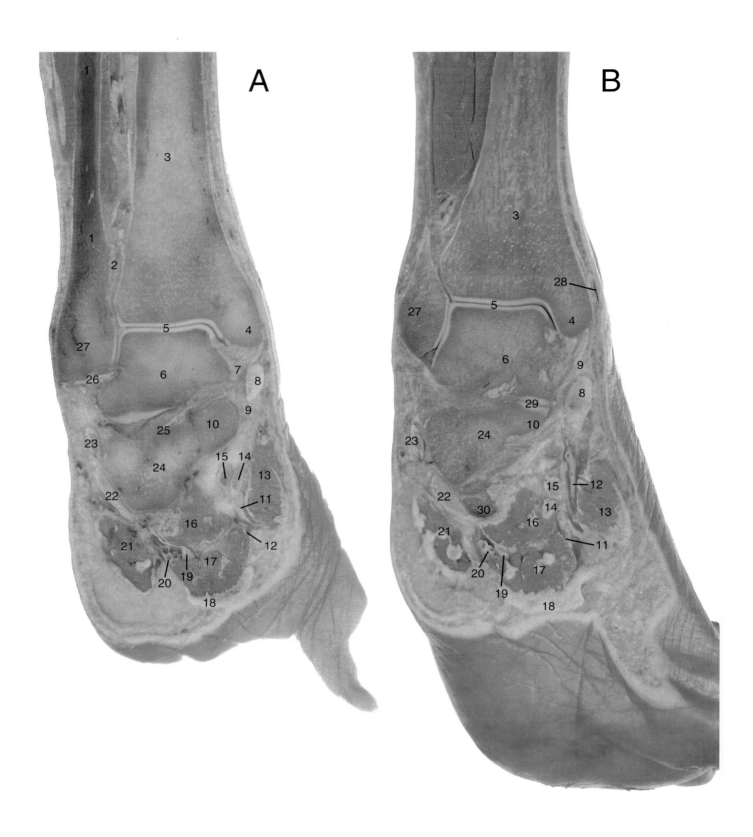

SECTIONS AND IMAGES OF THE FOOT
Coronal sections of the left ankle joint and foot (in plantarflexion)

A Through the posterior part of the talus, from behind

B About 1 cm in front of A, through the talocalcanean part of the talocalcaneonavicular joint, from behind

These coronal sections through the ankle joint (**5**) emphasize how the talus (**6**) is gripped between the two malleoli (**27** and **4**). In **A** the interosseous talocalcanean ligament (**25**) lies between the talus (**6**) and calcaneus (**24**), while in **B** the section has passed through the part of the sustentaculum tali (**10**) which forms the talocalcanean part of the talocalcaneonavicular joint (**29**). In the centre of the sole in both sections flexor digitorum brevis (**17**) overlies flexor accessorius (**16**); the fusion of accessorius with the tendon of flexor digitorum longus (**14**) is shown in **B**, where the tendon of flexor hallucis longus (**15**) has come to lie deep to the digitorum tendon (compare with the dissection **B** on page 79 and the section **B** on page 96).

1	Fibula
2	Interosseous tibiofibular ligament
3	Tibia
4	Medial malleolus
5	Ankle joint
6	Talus
7	Deep part of medial (deltoid) ligament
8	Tibialis posterior
9	Medial ligament
10	Sustentaculum tali
11	Medial plantar nerve
12	Medial plantar artery
13	Abductor hallucis
14	Flexor digitorum longus
15	Flexor hallucis longus
16	Flexor accessorius
17	Flexor digitorum brevis
18	Plantar aponeurosis
19	Lateral plantar nerve
20	Lateral plantar vessels
21	Abductor digiti minimi
22	Peroneus longus
23	Peroneus brevis
24	Calcaneus
25	Interosseous talocalcanean ligament
26	Posterior talofibular ligament
27	Lateral malleolus
28	Great saphenous vein
29	Talocalcanean part of talocalcaneonavicular joint
30	Cuboid

- **Joints, muscles and movements:**
  At the ankle joint
  Dorsiflexion: tibialis anterior, extensor hallucis longus, extensor digitorum longus, peroneus tertius
  Plantarflexion: gastrocnemius, soleus, plantaris, tibialis posterior, flexor hallucis longus, flexor digitorum longus.

  At the talocalcanean and talocalcaneonavicular joints
  Inversion: tibialis anterior and tibialis posterior.
  Eversion: peroneus longus, peroneus brevis and peroneus tertius.

- At the other small joints of the foot there are minor degrees of gliding or rotatory movements. At the transverse tarsal joint (page 47) a small amount of inversion and eversion occurs, but by far the greater part of these important movements takes place at the two joints beneath the talus. To visualize inversion and eversion, imagine the talus held firmly between the tibia and fibula, and the whole of the rest of the foot swivelling inwards or outwards underneath the talus. These movements do not take place at the ankle joint which essentially only allows dorsiflexion and plantarflexion.

- The actions of muscles on the toes are indicated by their names but the part played by the interossei and lumbricals requires some explanation (apart from the abduction and adduction produced by the interossei and referred to on page 81). Briefly the interossei and lumbricals work together to flex the metatarsophalangeal joints and extend the interphalangeal joints; these apparently contradictory actions on different joints by the same muscles can be explained as follows.

- The interossei (both plantar and dorsal) are attached mainly to the sides of the proximal phalanges but also into the dorsal digital expansions; the lumbricals are usually attached entirely to the expansions. Because of the position of these attachments in relation to the axis of movement of the metatarsophalangeal joints, the interossei and lumbricals plantarflex these joints.

- Because the lumbrical attachments and parts of the interosseus attachments are to the basal angles of the expansions, the line of pull is transmitted to the dorsal surfaces of the toes distal to the metatarsophalangeal joints, and so the interphalangeal joints are extended.

- In most feet the interosseus attachment to the expansion is minimal, and it is the lumbricals that are mainly responsible for assisting the long and short extensor tendons in extending the toes, keeping them straight and stabilized against the pull of the flexors which tend to make them buckle, especially during the push-off phase of walking when flexor hallucis longus and flexor digitorum longus are contracting strongly.

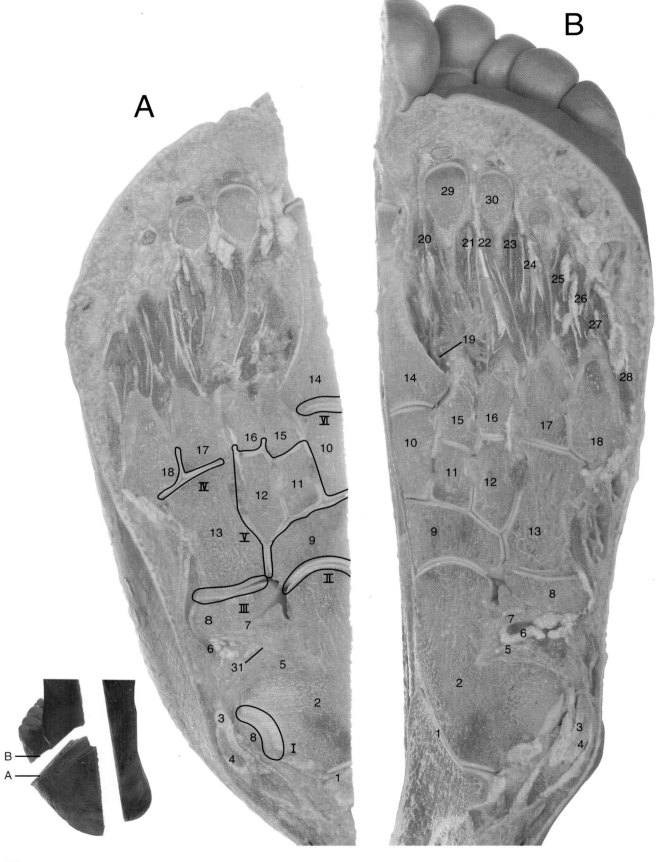

SECTIONS AND IMAGES OF THE FOOT
Oblique horizontal sections of the left foot

The plane of section is shown in the small illustration. The surfaces **A** and **B** have been separated and are viewed like two pages in an open book.

Between the tarsal bones in **A** the various joint cavities, outlined in black and numbered with Roman figures, are explained in the notes below.

In **B** the navicular (**9**) is seen between the talus (**2**) and the three cuneiforms (**10-12**). Note how the base of the second metatarsal (**15**) projects more proximally than the bases of the first and third metatarsals (**14** and **16**). On the lateral side the cuboid (**13**) articulates at the back with the very small part of the calcaneus (**8**) seen in this section, and at the front with the bases of the fourth and fifth metatarsals (**17** and **18**). Parts of all the interosseus muscles (four dorsal and three plantar, **20-26**) are identified in the forefoot.

1	Ankle joint
2	Talus
3	Peroneus brevis
4	Peroneus longus
5	Interosseous talocalcanean ligament
6	Extensor digitorum brevis
7	Cervical ligament
8	Calcaneus
9	Navicular
10	Medial ⎤
11	Intermediate ⎬ cuneiform
12	Lateral ⎦
13	Cuboid
14	First ⎤
15	Second ⎥
16	Third ⎬ metatarsal base
17	Fourth ⎥
18	Fifth ⎦
19	Deep plantar branch of first dorsal metatarsal artery
20	First dorsal ⎤
21	Second dorsal ⎥
22	First plantar ⎥
23	Third dorsal ⎬ interosseus
24	Second plantar ⎥
25	Fourth dorsal ⎥
26	Third plantar ⎦
27	Flexor digiti minimi brevis
28	Abductor digiti minimi
29	Head of second metatarsal
30	Head of third metatarsal
31	Inferior extensor retinaculum

- The cavities of a number of synovial joints in the foot are continuous with one another to the extent that there are normally six synovial cavities associated with the tarsal bones:

  I The talocalcanean joint cavity.

  II The talocalcaneonavicular joint cavity.

  III The calcaneocuboid joint cavity.

  IV The cuboideometatarsal joint cavity (between the cuboid and the bases of the fourth and fifth metatarsals).

  V The cuneonavicular and cuneometatarsal joint cavity (between the navicular, the three cuneiforms and the bases of the second, third and fourth metatarsals).

  VI The medial cuneometatarsal joint cavity (between the medial cuneiform and the base of the first metatarsal).

- Parts of all the above cavities can be seen in the foot sectioned here; they are indicated by the black lines in **A** and numbered as above. (The cuboideonavicular joint is usually a fibrous union but in this specimen it is synovial and continuous with the cuneonavicular joint cavity.)

SECTIONS AND IMAGES OF THE FOOT
Sections of the tarsus of the right foot
A Through the tranverse tarsal joint, proximal to the navicular
B Through the cuneonavicular joint, distal to the navicular

Both sections are viewed from behind, looking from the heel towards the toes

In **A** the section has passed through the talonavicular joint, so displaying the posterior (proximal) surface of the navicular (**7**). A small part of the cuboid (**8**) has been sliced off, leaving cartilage on the more lateral part of its posterior (calcanean) surface. The plantar aponeurosis (**14**) overlies flexor digitorum brevis (**15**), with abductor hallucis (**21**) on the medial side and abductor digiti minimi (**12**) laterally. Flexor accessorius

(**16**) lies centrally, with the tendons of flexor hallucis longus (**18**) and flexor digitorum longus (**19**) more medially placed at this level.

In **B** at the level of the posterior (navicular) surfaces of the cuneiform bones, the tendon of flexor hallucis longus (**18**) is now passing deep to the digitorum tendon (**19**). The tendon of peroneus longus (**11**) is turning laterally under the cuboid (**27**), where a little more distally it will become covered by the long plantar ligament (**29**) (compare with the dissection on page 85).

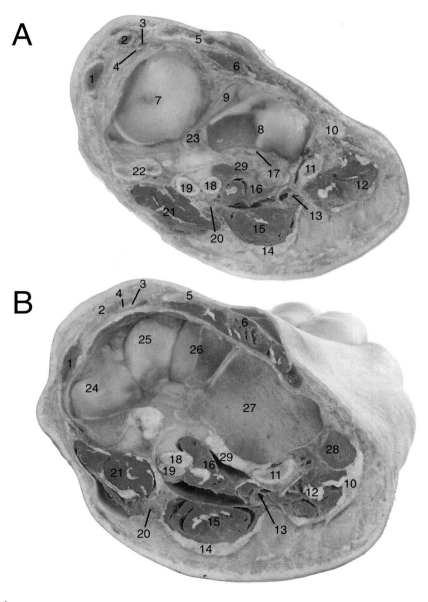

1	Tibialis anterior
2	Extensor hallucis longus
3	Dorsalis pedis artery
4	Deep peroneal nerve
5	Extensor digitorum longus
6	Extensor digitorum brevis
7	Posterior articular surface of navicular (for talus)
8	Posterior articular surface of cuboid (for calcaneus)
9	Anterior tip of calcaneus
10	Peroneus brevis
11	Peroneus longus
12	Abductor digiti minimi
13	Lateral plantar nerve and vessels
14	Plantar aponeurosis
15	Flexor digitorum brevis
16	Flexor accessorius
17	Plantar calcaneocuboid (short plantar) ligament
18	Flexor hallucis longus
19	Flexor digitorum longus
20	Medial plantar nerve and vessels
21	Abductor hallucis
22	Tibialis posterior
23	Plantar calcaneonavicular (spring) ligament
24	Medial ⎤
25	Intermediate ⎬ cuneiform
26	Lateral ⎦
27	Cuboid
28	Tuberosity of fifth metatarsal
29	Long plantar ligament

SECTIONS AND IMAGES OF THE FOOT
Sections of the right metatarsus
A Through the middle of the metatarsal shafts
B Through the heads of the first and fifth metatarsals

Both sections are viewed from behind, looking towards the toes. The metatarsals are numbered in Roman figures. On the dorsum the tendons of extensor digitorum longus to the appropriate toes are numbered **L2-L5**, and those of extensor digitorum brevis **B2-B4** (recall that the brevis tendon to the great toe is named extensor hallucis brevis, **2**). Similarly in the sole the flexor digitorum longus tendons are numbered **L2-L5**, with the

lumbrical muscles that arise from those tendons numbered **U1-U4**. The various interosseus muscles between and below the metatarsals have not been labelled.

In **B** note the sesamoid bones (**18**) under the head of the first metatarsal (**I**), with the tendon of flexor hallucis longus (**8**) between them.

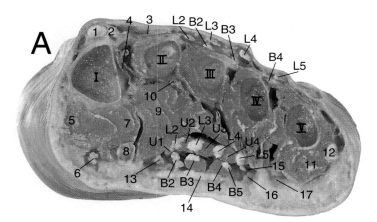

1	Extensor hallucis longus
2	Extensor hallucis brevis
3	Arcuate artery
4	Deep plantar artery
5	Abductor hallucis
6	Proper plantar digital nerve of great toe
7	Flexor hallucis brevis
8	Flexor hallucis longus
9	Oblique head of adductor hallucis
10	Second plantar metatarsal artery
11	Flexor digiti minimi brevis
12	Abductor digiti minimi
13	Common plantar digital branches of medial plantar nerve
14	Plantar aponeurosis
15	Deep branch of lateral plantar nerve
16	Fourth common plantar digital nerve
17	Proper plantar digital nerve of fifth toe
18	Sesamoid bone
19	Transverse head of adductor hallucis

GREAT TOE

The dorsum, nail, and sections of the great toe

A Dorsum of the right great toe
B Nail
C Nail bed of the left great toe
D Sagittal section of the right great toe, from the lateral side
E Coronal section of the distal phalanx of the right great toe

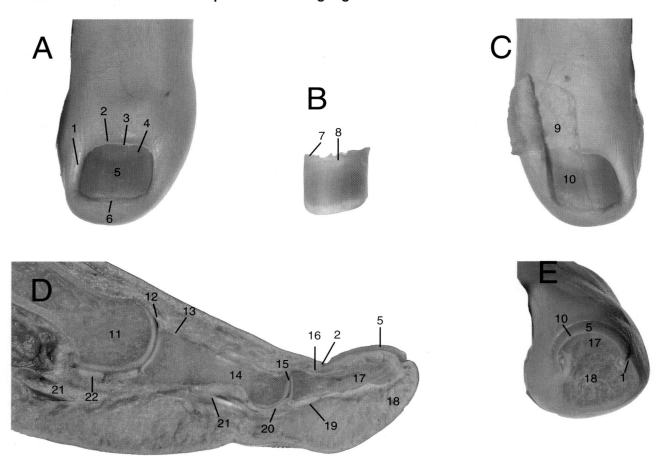

1 Nail wall	**12** Capsule of metatarsophalangeal joint
2 Nail fold	**13** Attachment of extensor hallucis brevis
3 Eponychium	**14** Proximal phalanx
4 Lunule ⎤	**15** Capsule of interphalangeal joint
5 Body	**16** Attachment of extensor hallucis longus
6 Free border ├ of nail	**17** Distal phalanx
7 Occult border	**18** Septa of pulp space
8 Root ⎦	**19** Attachment of flexor hallucis longus
9 Germinal matrix ⎤ of nail bed	**20** Plantar ligament of interphalangeal joint
10 Sterile matrix ⎦	**21** Flexor hallucis longus
11 Head of first metatarsal	**22** Sesamoid bone

RADIOGRAPHY OF THE FOOT
Radiographs
A From above (dorsoplantar view)
B Lateral view

The view in **A** looks down on to the dorsum of the right foot in front of the ankle, while the side view in **B** shows the ankle and other adjacent joints.

1 Calcaneus		**10** Proximal ⎤	
2 Head of talus		**11** Middle ⎬ phalanx of second toe	
3 Navicular		**12** Distal ⎦	
4 Cuboid		**13** Ankle joint	
5 Medial ⎤		**14** Talocalcanean joint	
6 Intermediate ⎬ cuneiform		**15** Calcaneocuboid joint	
7 Lateral ⎦		**16** Talonavicular part of ⎤ talocalcaneonavicular joint	
8 Second metatarsal		**17** Talocalcanean part of ⎦	
9 Sesamoid bone			

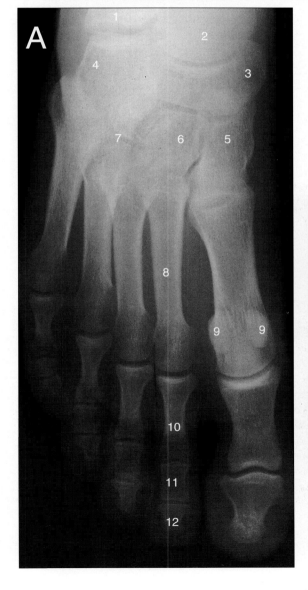

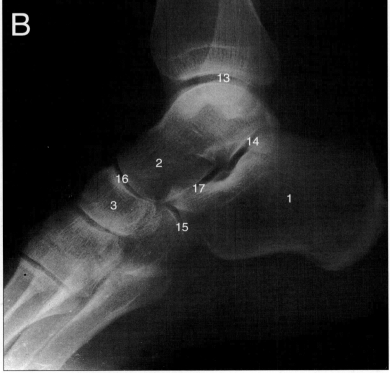

By courtesy of Dr Kate Stevens

RADIOGRAPHY OF THE FOOT
Ankle and foot joints
A Anteroposterior radiograph
B Lateral radiograph
C Radiograph standing on tip-toe
D Radiograph to show sesamoid bones under great toes

In **A** the talus (**5**) is embraced by the lateral and medial malleoli (**1** and **4**) and the lower end of the tibia, giving a very evenly-spaced ankle joint line (**3**).

The lateral view in **B** shows the tarsal sinus (**6**) between the talus and calcaneus, with the talocalcanean joint (**7**) behind the sinus and the talocalcanean part (**9**) of the talocalcaneonavicular joint in front of it. The talonavicular part of the talocalcaneonavicular joint is in front of the head of the talus (**8**). Behind the cuboid (**13**) is the calcaneocuboid joint (**12**), and in front of it the articulations with the fourth and fifth metatarsals (**15** and **16**). Below the cuboid is a small (occasional) sesamoid bone in the tendon of peroneus longus (**14**).

Compare the metatarsals and sesamoid bones in **C** and **D** with those on page 40

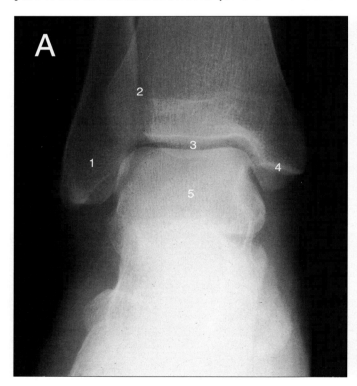

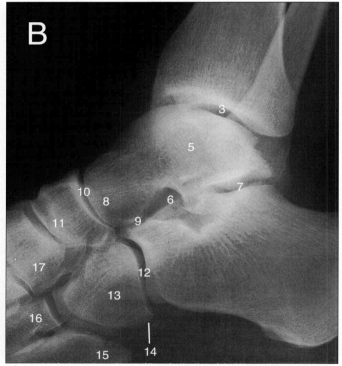

By courtesy of Dr Kate Stevens

1 Lateral malleolus	**11** Navicular bone
2 Inferior tibiofibular joint	**12** Calcaneocuboid joint
3 Ankle joint	**13** Cuboid bone
4 Medial malleolus	**14** Sesamoid bone in tendon of peroneus longus
5 Talus	**15** Tuberosity of base of fifth metatarsal
6 Tarsal sinus	**16** Base of fourth metatarsal
7 Talocalcanean joint	**17** Cuneiform bones
8 Head of talus	
9 Talocalcanean part ⎤ of talocalcaneonavicular	
10 Talonavicular part ⎦ joint	

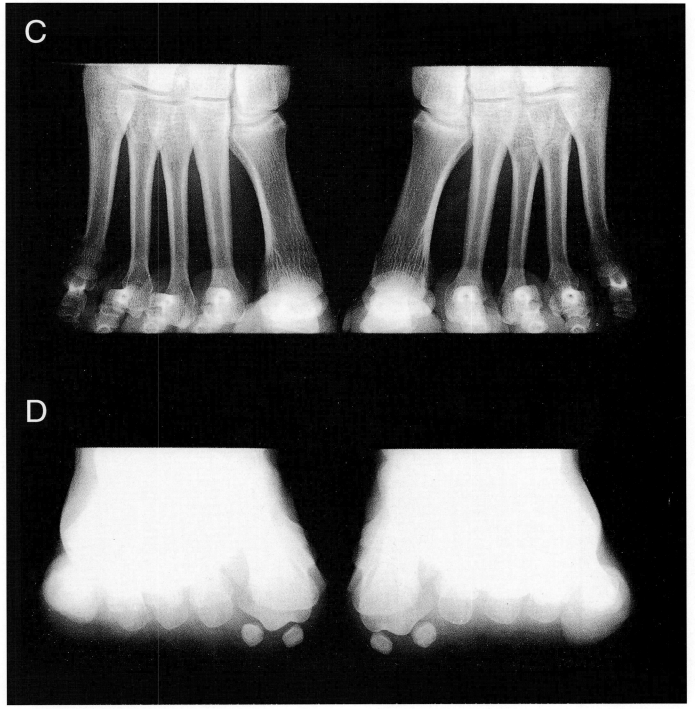

By courtesy of Mr W. Stripp

APPENDIX
MUSCLES

MUSCLES OF THE GLUTEAL REGION

Gluteus maximus
From the posterior gluteal line of the hip bone, the dorsal surface of the lower part of the sacrum and the side of the coccyx, the sacrotuberous ligament, and the fascia over gluteus medius
To the iliotibial tract, with the deep fibres of the lower part attaching to the gluteal tuberosity of the femur
Inferior gluteal nerve, L5, S1, 2
Extension and lateral rotation of the hip joint

Gluteus medius
From the outer surface of the ilium between the posterior and anterior oblique lines
To the lateral surface of the greater trochanter of the femur
Superior gluteal nerve, L4, 5, S1
Abduction and medial rotation of the hip joint, and prevention of adduction

Gluteus minimus
From the outer surface of the ilium between the anterior and inferior gluteal lines
To the anterior part of the lateral surface of the greater trochanter of the femur
Superior gluteal nerve, L4, 5, S1
Abduction and medial rotation of the hip joint, and prevention of adduction

Piriformis
From the middle three pieces of the sacrum
To the upper border of the greater trochanter of the femur
Branches from L5, S1, 2
Abduction, lateral rotation and stabilization of the hip joint

Quadratus femoris
From the upper part of the outer border of the ischial tuberosity
To the quadrate tubercle of the intertrochanteric crest of the femur
Nerve to quadratus femoris, L4, 5, S1
Lateral rotation and stabilization of the hip joint

Obturator internus
From the inner surface of the obturator membrane and the adjacent anterolateral pelvic wall
To the greater trochanter of the femur, above and in front of the trochanteric fossa
Nerve to obturator internus, L5, S1, 2
Lateral rotation and stabilization of the hip joint

Gemellus superior and inferior
Superior from the dorsal surface of the ischial spine, inferior from the upper part of the ischial tuberosity
To the superior and inferior borders respectively of obturator internus
Nerves to obturator internus (superior) and quadratus femoris (inferior)
Assists obturator internus

Obturator externus
From the outer surface of the obturator membrane and the ischiopubic ramus
To the trochanteric fossa of the femur
Obturator nerve, L3, 4,
Lateral rotator of the thigh

MUSCLES OF THE FRONT OF THE THIGH

Iliacus
From the upper two-thirds of the iliac fossa in the lower abdomen
To the psoas tendon and the femur below and in front of the lesser trochanter
Femoral nerve, L2, 3
Flexor of the hip, assisting psoas major

Psoas major
From the sides of the lumbar vertebrae and intervertebral discs
To the lesser trochanter of the femur
Branches from L1, 2, 3
Flexor of the hip

Tensor fasciae latae
From the anterior 5 cm of the outer lip of the iliac crest
To the iliotibial tract
Superior gluteal nerve, L4, 5, S1
Extensor of the knee and lateral rotator of the leg

Sartorius
From the anterior superior iliac spine
To the upper part of the medial surface of the shaft of the tibia in front of gracilis and semitendinosus
Femoral nerve, L2, 3
Flexor, adductor and lateral rotator of the hip

Rectus femoris
From the anterior inferior iliac spine (straight head) and the ilium above the rim of the acetabulum (reflected head)

To the base of the patella
Femoral nerve, L3, 4
Flexor of the hip and extensor of the knee

Vastus lateralis
From the upper part of the intertrochanteric line of
the femur, anterior and inferior borders of the
greater trochanter, lateral lip of the gluteal
tuberosity and the upper part of the linea aspera
To the lateral border of the patella and the
quadriceps tendon
Femoral nerve, L2, 3, 4
Extensor of the knee

Vastus medialis
From the lower part of the intertrochanteric line of
the femur, the spiral line, the linea aspera, the
upper part of the medial supracondylar line and
the tendon of adductor magnus
To the medial border of the patella and the
quadriceps tendon
Femoral nerve, L2, 3, 4
Extensor of the knee

Vastus intermedius
From the anterior and lateral surfaces of the upper
two-thirds of the shaft of the femur
To the deep part of the quadriceps tendon
Femoral nerve, L2, 3, 4
Extensor of the knee

Articularis genu
From the anterior surface of the femur below vastus
intermedius
To the apex of the suprapatellar bursa
Femoral nerve, L3, 4
Retraction of the bursa as the knee extends

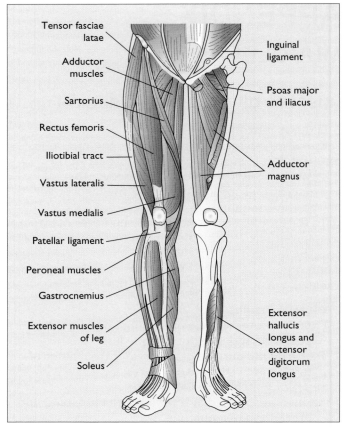

Fig. 1 Muscles: From the front. Superficial muscles on the
right side of the body; deep muscles on the left side.

MUSCLES OF THE MEDIAL SIDE OF THE THIGH

Pectineus
From the pectineal line of the pubis and bone in
front of the line
To the femur on a line from the lesser trochanter to
the linea aspera
Femoral nerve, L2, 3
Flexor, adductor and lateral rotator of the hip

Gracilis
From the body of the pubis and ischiopubic ramus
To the upper part of the medial surface of the shaft
of the tibia, between sartorius and
semitendinosus
Obturator nerve, L2, 3
Flexor, adductor and medial rotator of the thigh

Adductor brevis
From the body and inferior ramus of the pubis
To the shaft of the femur on a line from the lesser
trochanter to the linea aspera, and to the upper
part of the linea
Obturator nerve, L2, 3, 4
Adductor of the thigh

Adductor longus
From the front of the pubis
To the middle part of the linea aspera
Obturator nerve, L2, 3, 4
Adductor of the thigh

Adductor magnus

From the lower lateral part of the ischial tuberosity and the ischiopubic ramus

To the shaft of the femur from the gluteal tuberosity along the linea aspera to the medial supracondylar line, and to the adductor tubercle

Obturator nerve, L2, 3, 4 and sciatic nerve, L4, 5, S1

Adductor and lateral rotator of the thigh

MUSCLES OF THE BACK OF THE THIGH

Biceps femoris

From the medial facet of the ischial tuberosity with semimembranosus (long head) and from the linea aspera and lateral supracondylar line of the femur (short head)

To the head of the fibula

Sciatic nerve (tibial part to long head, common peroneal part to short head), L5, S1

Flexion and lateral rotation of the knee and extension of the hip

Semitendinosus

From the medial facet of the ischial tubosity, with the long head of biceps

To the upper part of the subcutaneous surface of the tibia, behind gracilis

Sciatic nerve (tibial part), L5, S1

Flexion and medial rotation of the knee, and extension of the hip

Semimembranosus

From the lateral facet of the ischial tuberosity

To the groove on the back of the medial condyle of the tibia, with expansions forming the oblique popliteal ligament and the fascia over popliteus

Sciatic nerve (tibial part), L5, S1

Flexion and medial rotation of the knee, and extension of the hip

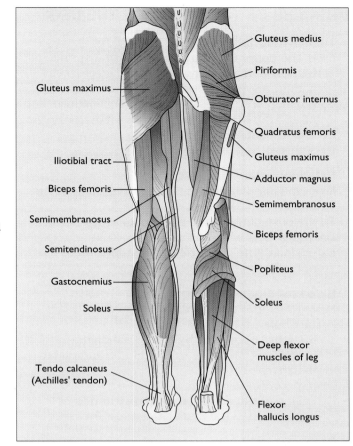

Fig. 2 Muscles: From the back. Superficial muscles on the left side of the body; deep muscles on the right side.

MUSCLES OF THE FRONT OF THE LEG

Tibialis anterior
From the upper two-thirds of the lateral surface of the tibia and adjoining part of the interosseus membrane
To the medial surfaces of the medial cuneiform and base of the first metatarsal
Deep peroneal nerve, L4, 5
Dorsiflexion and inversion of the foot

Extensor hallucis longus
From the middle third of the medial surface of the fibula
To the base of the distal phalanx of the great toe
Deep peroneal nerve, L4, 5
Extension of the great toe and dorsiflexion of the foot

Extensor digitorum longus
From the upper two-thirds of the medial surface of the fibula
To the four lateral toes by the dorsal digital expansions, attached to the middle and distal phalanges
Deep peroneal nerve, L5, S1
Extension of the second to fifth toes and dorsiflexion of the foot

Peroneus tertius
From the lower third of the medial surface of the fibula, continuous with extensor digitorum longus
To the shaft of the fifth metatarsal
Deep peroneal nerve, L5, S1
Dorsiflexion and eversion of the foot

MUSCLE OF THE DORSUM OF THE FOOT

Extensor digitorum brevis
From the upper surface of the calcaneus
To the base of the proximal phalanx of the great toe (as extensor hallucis brevis) and the dorsal digital expansions of the second to fourth toes
Deep peroneal nerve, L5, S1
Extension of the first to fourth toes

MUSCLES OF THE LATERAL SIDE OF THE LEG

Peroneus longus
From the upper two-thirds of the lateral surface of the fibula
To the lateral sides of the medial cuneiform and base of the first metatarsal
Superficial peroneal nerve, L5, S1, 2
Plantarflexion and eversion of the foot

Peroneus brevis
From the lower two-thirds of the lateral surface of the fibula
To the tuberosity of the base of the fifth metatarsal
Superficial peroneal nerve, L5, S1, 2
Plantarflexion and eversion of the foot

MUSCLES OF THE BACK OF THE LEG

Gastrocnemius
Medial head from the upper posterior part of the medial condyle of the femur; lateral head from the lateral surface of the lateral condyle of the femur
To the middle of the posterior surface of the calcaneus by the tendo calcaneus (in association with soleus)
Tibial nerve, S1, 2
Plantarflexion of the foot and flexion of the knee

Soleus
From the soleal line and upper part of the medial border of the tibia, a tendinous arch over the popliteal vessels and tibial nerve, and the upper part of the posterior surface of the fibula
To the tendo calcaneus with gastrocnemius (see above)
Tibial nerve, S1, 2
Plantarflexion of the foot

Plantaris
From the lateral supracondylar line of the femur
To the calcaneus on the medial side of the tendo calcaneus
Tibial nerve, S1, 2
Plantarflexion of the foot and weak flexion of the knee

Popliteus
From the back of the tibia above the soleal line
To the outer surface of the lateral epicondyle of the femur
Tibial nerve, L4, 5, S1
Lateral rotation of the femur on the fixed tibia (or medial rotation of the tibia on the fixed femur); pulls lateral meniscus backwards during flexion of the knee

Tibialis posterior
From the posterior surface of the interosseous membrane and adjacent posterior surfaces of the tibia and fibula
To the tuberosity of the navicular, with slips to other tarsal bones (except the talus) and the middle three metatarsals
Tibial nerve, L4, 5
Plantarflexion and inversion of the foot

Flexor hallucis longus
From the lower two-thirds of the posterior surface of the fibula
To the plantar surface of the base of the distal phalanx of the great toe
Tibial nerve, S2, 3
Plantarflexion of the great toe and foot

Flexor digitorum longus
From the medial part of the posterior surface of the tibia below the soleal line
To the four lateral toes by a tendon to each, reaching the plantar surface of the base of the distal phalanx
Tibial nerve, S2, 3
Plantarflexion of the four lateral toes and foot

MUSCLES OF THE SOLE OF THE FOOT

FIRST LAYER

Abductor hallucis
From the medial process of the calcanean
   tuberosity and the plantar aponeurosis
To the medial side of the proximal phalanx of the
   great toe
Medial plantar nerve, S2, 3
Abduction and plantarflexion of the great toe

Flexor digitorum brevis
From the medial process of the calcanean
   tuberosity and the deep surface of the central
   part of the plantar aponeurosis
To the lateral four toes by a tendon to each; the
   tendon divides into two slips (to allow the flexor
   digitorum longus tendon to pass between them)
   which are attached to the sides of the middle
   phalanx
Medial plantar nerve, S2, 3
Plantarflexion of the four lateral toes

Abductor digiti minimi
From the lateral and medial processes of the
   calcanean tuberosity and the plantar aponeurosis
To the lateral side of the base of the proximal phalanx
   of the fifth toe (with flexor digiti minimi brevis)
Lateral plantar nerve, S2, 3
Abduction and plantarflexion of the fifth toe

SECOND LAYER

Flexor accessorius (quadratus plantae)
From the (concave) medial surface of the calcaneus
   and from the plantar surface of the calcaneus in
   front of the lateral process of the tuberosity
To the lateral border of flexor digitorum longus
   before the division into four tendons
Lateral plantar nerve, S2, 3
Assistance with plantarflexion of the four lateral
   toes

Lumbricals
First lumbrical from the medial border of the first
   tendon of flexor digitorum longus
Second, third and fourth lumbricals from the four
   adjoining tendons of flexor digitorum longus
To the medial sides of the dorsal digital expansions
   of the tendons of extensor digitorum longus
First lumbrical - medial plantar nerve; second, third
   and fourth lumbrical by the lateral plantar nerve,
   S2, 3
Plantarflexion at the four lateral metatarsophalan-
   geal joints and extension at interphalangeal joints

Tendons of flexor digitorum longus and flexor
   hallucis longus

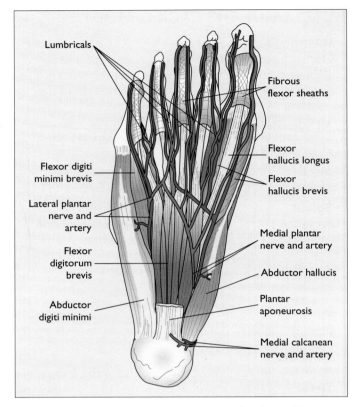

Fig 3 Muscles of the sole of the right foot: first layer. For
dissection see page 78.

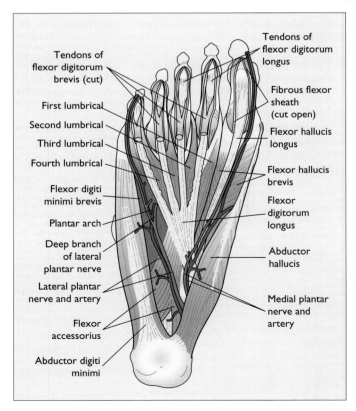

Fig 4 Muscles of the sole of the right foot: second layer. For
dissection see page 79.

THIRD LAYER

Flexor hallucis brevis

From the plantar surface of the cuboid and lateral cuneiform

By a tendon to each side of the base of the proximal phalanx of the great toe, the medial tendon joining with that of abductor hallucis and the lateral with adductor hallucis; there is a sesamoid bone in each tendon

Medial plantar nerve, S2, 3

Plantarflexion of the metatarsophalangeal joint of the great toe

Adductor hallucis

Oblique head from the bases of the second, third and fourth metatarsals

Transverse head from the plantar metatarsophalangeal ligaments of the third, fourth and fifth toes

To the lateral side of the base of the proximal phalanx of the great toe, with part of flexor hallucis brevis

Lateral plantar nerve, S2, 3

Adduction of the great toe

Flexor digiti minimi brevis

From the plantar surface of the base of the fifth metatarsal

To the lateral side of the base of proximal phalanx of the fifth toe, with abductor digiti minimi

Lateral plantar nerve, S2, 3

Plantarflexion of the metatarsophalangeal joint of the fifth toe

FOURTH LAYER

Dorsal interosseus (four)

From adjacent sides of the bodies of the metatarsals

To the bases of proximal phalanges and the dorsal digital expansions. First and second to the medial and lateral sides of the second toe; third and fourth to the lateral sides of the third and fourth toes

Lateral plantar nerve, S2, 3

Plantarflexion of the metatarsophalangeal joints and extension (dorsiflexion) of the interphalangeal joints of the second, third and fourth toes; abduction of the same toes

Plantar interosseus (three)

From the bases and medial sides of the third, fourth and fifth metatarsals

To the medial sides of the bases of the proximal phalanges and dorsal digital expansions of the corresponding toes

Lateral plantar nerve, S2, 3

Plantarflexion of the metatarsophalangeal joints and extension (dorsiflexion) of the interphalangeal joints of the third, fourth and fifth toes; adduction of the same toes

Tendons of tibialis posterior and peroneus longus

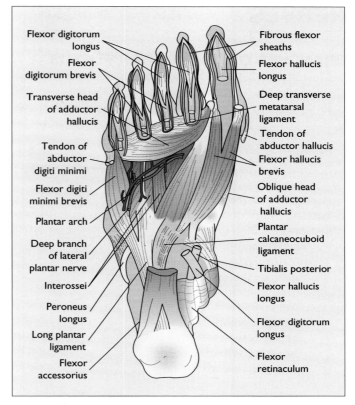

Fig 5 Muscles of the sole of the right foot: third layer. For dissection see page 80.

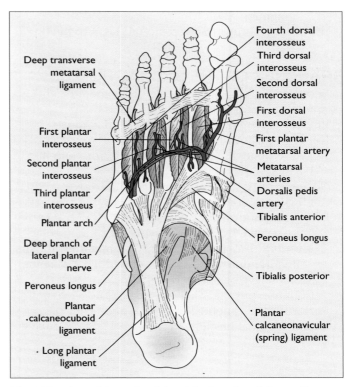

Fig 6 Muscles of the sole of the right foot: fourth layer. For dissection see page 81.

NERVES

BRANCHES OF THE LUMBAR PLEXUS

Muscular T12, L1, 2, 3, 4 to psoas major and minor, quadratus lumborum and iliacus

Iliohypogastric and ilio-inguinal L1 to parts of internal oblique and transversus abdominis in anterior abdominal wall

Genitofemoral L1, 2, giving off
    Genital branch (to cremaster muscle of spermatic cord)
    Femoral branch

Lateral cutaneous of thigh L2, 3

Femoral L2, 3, 4, giving off
    Nerve to pectineus
    Anterior division, giving off
        Intermediate femoral cutaneous
        Medial femoral cutaneous
        Nerve to sartorius
    Posterior division, giving off
        Saphenous
        Nerves to quadriceps femoris

Obturator L2, 3, 4, giving off
    Anterior branch
        Muscular to adductor longus, adductor brevis and gracilis
    Posterior branch
        Muscular to obturator externus and adductor magnus

Accessory obturator (occasional) L3, 4 to pectineus

BRANCHES OF THE SACRAL PLEXUS

Superior gluteal L4, 5, S1, to gluteus medius, gluteus minimus and tensor fasciae latae

Inferior gluteal L5, S1, 2, to gluteus maximus

Nerve to piriformis S1, 2

Nerve to quadratus femoris and inferior gemellus L4, 5, S1

Nerve to obturator internus and superior gemellus L5, S1, 2

Posterior femoral cutaneous S2, 3

Sciatic nerve L4, 5, S1, 2, 3 giving off
    Muscular branches to biceps, semimembranosus, semitendinosus and part of adductor magnus
    Tibial nerve - see below
    Common peroneal nerve – see below

Perforating cutaneous, pudendal and other pelvic and perineal branches

BRANCHES OF THE TIBIAL NERVE L4, 5, S1, 2, 3

Muscular to gastrocnemius, plantaris, soleus, popliteus, tibialis posterior, flexor digitorum longus and flexor hallucis longus

Sural (ending as lateral dorsal cutaneous and then dorsal digital to lateral side of fifth toe)

Medial calcanean

Medial plantar – see below

Lateral plantar – see below

BRANCHES OF THE COMMON PERONEAL NERVE L4, 5, S1, 2

Recurrent

Lateral cutaneous of calf

Peroneal communicating

Superficial peroneal, giving off
    Muscular to peroneus longus and peroneus brevis
    Medial branch (medial dorsal cutaneous), giving off
        Dorsal digital
    Lateral branch (intermediate dorsal cutaneous), giving off
        Dorsal digital

Deep peroneal, giving off
    Muscular to tibialis anterior, extensor hallucis longus, externsor digitorum longus and peroneus tertius
    Lateral terminal, to extensor digitorum brevis
    Medial terminal, giving off
        Dorsal digital (to first cleft)

BRANCHES OF THE MEDIAL PLANTAR NERVE L4, 5, S1

Trunk giving off
    Nerve to abductor hallucis
    Nerve to flexor digitorum brevis,

Proper plantar digital nerve of great toe, giving off
    Nerve to flexor hallucis brevis.

First common plantar digital nerve, giving off
    Nerve to first lumbrical
    Proper plantar digital nerves of first cleft

Second common plantar digital nerve, giving off
    Proper plantar digital nerves of second cleft

Third common plantar digital nerve, giving off
    Proper plantar digital nerves of third cleft.

BRANCHES OF THE LATERAL PLANTAR NERVE S1, 2

Trunk, giving off
    Nerve to flexor accessorius
    Nerve to abductor digiti minimi
Superficial branch, giving off
    Fourth common plantar digital nerve, giving off
        Proper plantar digital nerves of fourth cleft
    Proper plantar digital nerve of fifth toe, giving off
    Nerve to flexor digiti minimi brevis
    Nerve to third plantar interosseus
    Nerve to fourth dorsal interosseus
Deep branch, giving off
    Nerve to adductor hallucis
    Nerves to second, third and fourth lumbricals
    Nerves to first, second and third dorsal interossei
    Nerves to first and second plantar interossei.

REGIONAL ANAESTHESIA OF THE FOOT

For operations on the front part of the foot, one or more of the five nerves that supply the foot – tibial, saphenous, superficial peroneal, deep peroneal, and sural – can be infiltrated with local anaesthetic. The object is to deliver the solution adjacent to the nerve trunks so that it can diffuse into them from the surrounding tissue; the nerves themselves must not be penetrated by the needle. In all cases before injection of the anaesthetic solution, aspiration must be attempted to ensure that the needle tip has not entered a blood vessel.

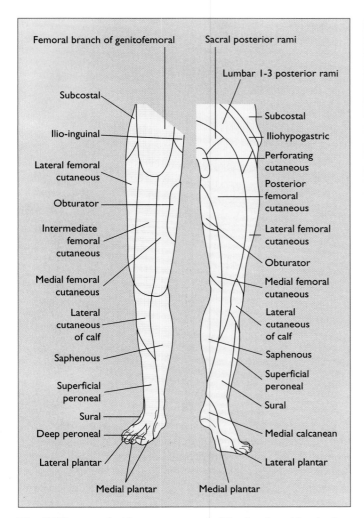

Fig. 7 Diagram of cutaneous nerves of the front and back of the right lower limb.

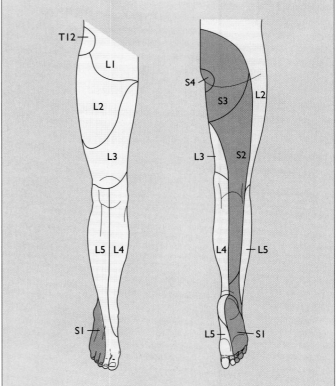

Fig. 8 Diagram of dermatomes of the front and back of the right lower limb. (A dermatome is the area of skin supplied by any one spinal nerve.) Note that both the dorsum and sole of the foot are supplied by L5 and S1 dermatomes.

Tibial nerve

For infiltration of the tibial nerve behind the medial malleolus (page 73), the needle is inserted at the medial edge of the Achilles' tendon, 2 cm above the tip of the medial malleolus and at right angles to the tibia. The needle is advanced until it touches the tibia and is then withdrawn slightly; the object is to allow the solution to percolate into the neurovascular compartment deep to the flexor retinaculum.

Saphenous and superficial peroneal nerves

The saphenous and superficial peroneal nerves can be infiltrated as they approach the dorsum of the foot between the two malleoli (page 64). The needle is inserted in front of the medial malleolus and is directed transversely and subcutaneously towards the lateral malleolus, deep to the superficial veins but superficial to the extensor tendons.

Deep peroneal nerve

The deep peroneal nerve can be infiltrated at the level of the middle of the tarsus as it lies between the tendon of extensor hallucis longus and the second toe tendon of extensor digitorum longus (page 74). The needle is inserted perpendicular to the dorsum, between the tendons and lateral to the dorsalis pedis artery (if present and palpable), so that the solution infiltrates the tissues over the first intermetatarsal space.

Sural nerve

The sural nerve can be infiltrated above and behind the tip of the lateral malleolus by a needle inserted lateral to the Achilles' tendon and directed perpendicularly towards the peroneus longus tendon, avoiding the small saphenous vein (page 67).

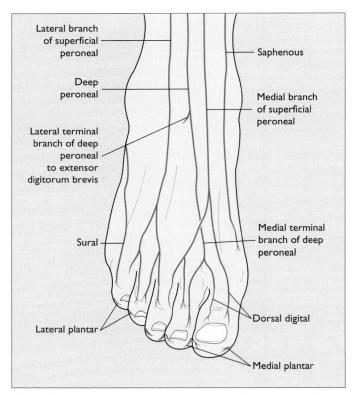

Fig. 9 Diagram of nerves of the dorsum of the right foot. Note that the tips of the toes are supplied from the sole by digital branches of the medial and lateral plantar nerves; their terminations curl round on to the dorsum of the toes in the region of the nails.

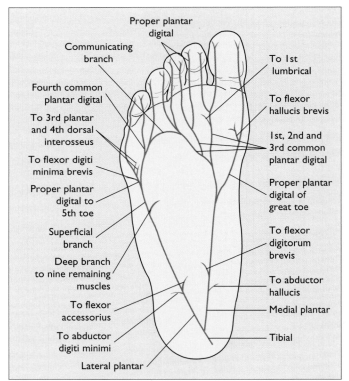

Fig. 10 Diagram of branches of the right medial and lateral plantar nerves. The medial plantar nerve gives off branches to four of the muscles of the sole (abductor hallucis, flexor digitorum brevis, flexor hallucis brevis and the first lumbrical); all the other muscles of the sole are supplied by the lateral plantar nerve (see the notes on page 74). Often, as shown here, there is a communicating branch between the adjacent plantar digital branches of the medial and lateral plantar nerves.

ARTERIES

BRANCHES OF THE FEMORAL ARTERY

Giving off the following before becoming the
    popliteal artery
Superficial epigastric
Superficial circumflex iliac
Superficial external pudendal
Deep external pudendal
Profunda femoris, giving off
    Lateral circumflex femoral
    Medial circumflex femoral
    Perforating
Descending genicular

BRANCHES OF THE POPLITEAL ARTERY

Sural
Superior, middle and inferior genicular
Anterior tibial, giving off the following before
    becoming the dorsalis pedis artery (see below)
    Posterior and anterior tibial recurrent
    Anterior medial and anterior lateral malleolar
Posterior tibial, giving off
    Circumflex fibular
    Peroneal, giving off
        Nutrient to the fibula
        Perforating
        Communicating
        Lateral malleolar
        Calcanean
    Nutrient to the tibia
    Communicating
    Medial malleolar
    Calcanean
    Medial plantar – see below
    Lareral plantar – see below

BRANCHES OF THE DORSALIS PEDIS ARTERY

Lateral tarsal
Medial tarsal
First dorsal metatarsal, giving off
    Deep plantar (perforating) branch, to complete
        plantar arch
    Dorsal digital branch to medial side of great toe
    Dorsal digital branches of first cleft
Arcuate, giving off
    Second dorsal metatarsal, giving off
        Perforating branches
        Dorsal digital branches to second cleft
    Third dorsal metatarsal, giving off
        Perforating branches
        Dorsal digital branches to third cleft
    Fourth dorsal metatarsal, giving off
        Perforating branches
        Dorsal digital branches to fourth cleft
        Dorsal digital branch to lateral side of fifth toe.

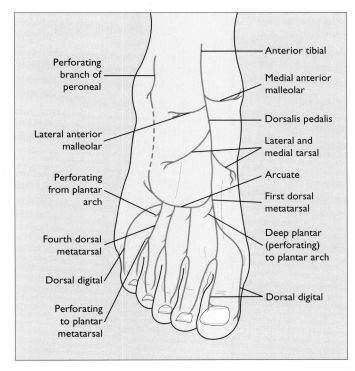

Fig. 11 Diagram of branches of the right dorsalis pedis artery, excluding muscular and most anastomotic branches, but note that anastomoses from the perforating branch of the peroneal artery may link up with the arcuate artery and enlarge to replace an absent dorsalis pedis artery.

BRANCHES OF THE MEDIAL PLANTAR ARTERY

Anastomotic branch to plantar digital artery of medial side of the great toe

Superficial digital branches to anastomose with first, second and third plantar metatarsal arteries.

BRANCHES OF THE LATERAL PLANTAR ARTERY

Plantar arch, giving off
    First plantar metatarsal, giving off
        Plantar digital artery to medial side of great toe
        Plantar digital arteries to first cleft
    Second, third and fourth plantar metatarsal arteries, each giving off
        Plantar digital arteries to second, third and fourth clefts respectively
    Perforating branches
Plantar digital artery to lateral side of fifth toe.

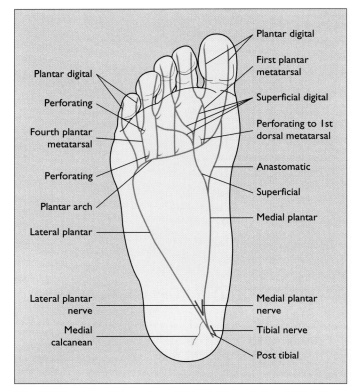

Fig. 12 Diagram of branches of the right medial and lateral plantar arteries (excluding muscular and most anastomotic branches). The proximal parts of the medial and lateral plantar nerves are shown in green to indicate that the nerves lie on the internal sides of their corresponding arteries.

Index

Page numbers refer to items in the text as well as those illustrated.

118

- lateral of talus 41, 48, 88
- medial of talus 48
Tuberosity of calcaneus 34, 36, 45, 58, 77, 87, 88
- of cuboid bone 60
- of fifth metatarsal 34, 36, 41, 62, 82, 85, 96
- ischial 18, 19, 23
- of navicular bone 34, 36, 41, 44, 60, 80, 81, 84, 85, 90
- of tibia 16, 26, 30

Upper limb 45

Valves of veins 66
Vein(s), accessory saphenous 22
- anterior tibial 69
- dorsal arch 34, 64, 66, 67
- dorsal digital 66
- dorsal metatarsal 66
- femoral 15, 23
- great saphenous 10, 14, 22, 23, 32, 34, 64, 66, 76, 90, 92
- marginal 66, 67
- perforating 64–67
- popliteal 30–32
- posterior arch 65, 66
- posterior tibial 71, 72
- small saphenous 12, 30, 32, 34, 36, 65, 66

- superficial epigastric 22
- varicose 66
- *see also* Artery
Venae comitantes 71, 72, 75
Vessel(s), anterior tibial 74, 90
- dorsalis pedis 69
- femoral 22, 25
- lateral malleolar 74
- lateral plantar 78, 86–88, 90–92, 96
- lateral tarsal 74
- lymph 66
- medial circumflex femoral 20
- medial plantar 78, 86, 87, 90, 96
- peroneal 90
- popliteal 31
- profunda femoris 25
- superficial 64–67
- superficial circumflex iliac 22
- superficial external pudendal 22
- *see also* Artery, Vein
Vinculum, long 80

Walking 45, 93
Weight, weight-bearing 35, 45, 77